BEYOND BIRTH TRAUMA
THE ROAD TO HEALING

Emma Jane Cushnan

CHAPTERS

DEDICATION

To everyone who made this possible, who showed me that there was hope and light. That told me I was more than what happened to me. That helped me believe I could break free from the darkness of my cocoon, find my wings again so I could soar beyond birth trauma and then in turn help others.

To those who showed me, it was ok to be broken, who helped me fill the cracks in my soul and heal with their love and support.

To the brave courageous ones who battle the endless fight of birth trauma not knowing how brave and strong they are. Who through eyes of sorrow miss how they shine such incredible blinding light into the lives of others.

To my husband, the love of my life, who helped me believe that this book was possible, who encouraged me, inspired me and supported me on my journey to healing. You are my constant, my anchor in life's stormy seas, my soulmate.

To my two beautiful daughters Kathryn and Alisha for your love, support and encouragement. This journey has been for you, to make this world a better more caring place, a world of hope. You are, always have been, and will always be, my world. I love you.

'May your scars be the wings that carry you into the glorious light.'

Love Emma Jane X

THE BIRTH TRAUMA TREE

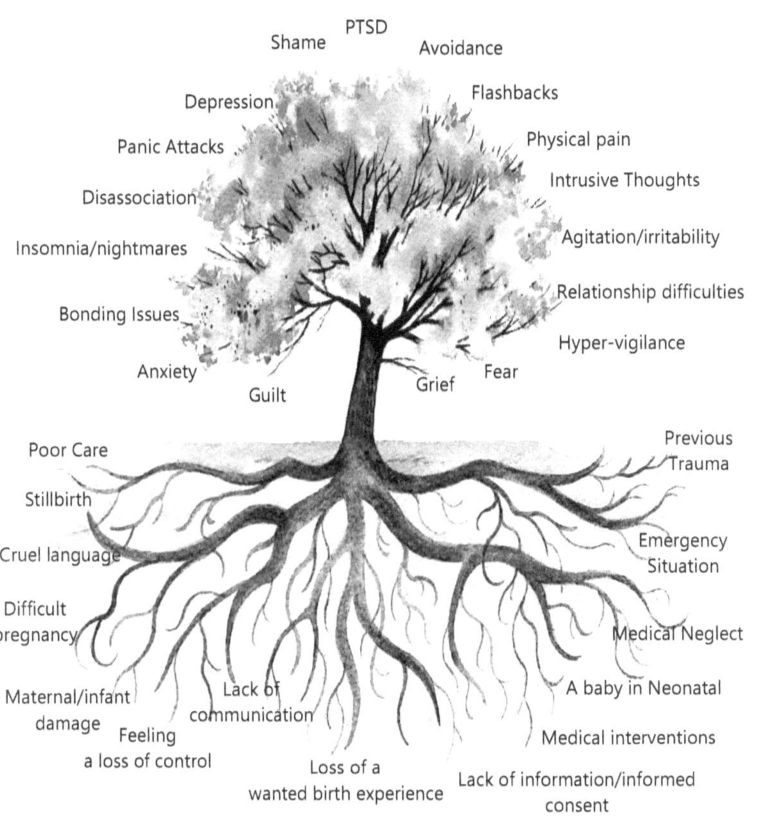

POEM

Every day is a battle she believes she cannot win.
Behind her smile, she hides the pain that lies deep within.

She searches for her new beginning, trying hard to let go
of the past.
She dreams of calmer, happy days and good times that will
last.

While she sees only darkness, around her dances light.
Worn down by the inner warring but never giving up the
fight.

As fragile as a butterfly she sometimes appears to be.
Yet her strength makes her wings unfold, her true beauty
for all to see.

Inside the voices churn and quarrel, making her worry and
doubt.
Yet those that love and need her, never go without.

Despite the silent torment that leaves her feeling bare.
She envelopes others in her love, there's always plenty to
spare.

She doesn't always believe that she's needed by one and all.
Always in her heart, she fears she may stumble and fall.

So, each night hold her against your beating heart,
and hope one day she realises she's your whole world, yes
every part.

"Following birth trauma, I felt I was stumbling around in the dark not knowing where to go for support. The effects of birth trauma caused me incredible pain both physically and emotionally. I came across Emma and she made me feel seen, included and safe. Emma has supported me for many years now, trauma never goes away but its effects are lessened when you have wonderful people to turn to.

For me, Emma was that person. She always had time to listen, to show love and understanding. Emma is a beautiful soul, and without her, I would be lost. I would go as far as to say that Emma saved my life and I will be eternally grateful to her. I'm so glad I get to call Emma my friend."

Claire
(Midwife and Mother)

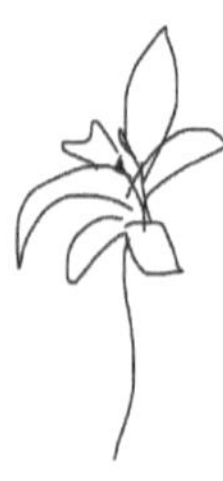

A LITTLE ABOUT ME

Hello, I'm Emma Jane. I'm a mother to two wonderful daughters who fill my life with happiness, vibrancy, love and plenty of surprises. I'm lucky to live in the beautiful Welsh countryside with my wonderful husband.

Sadly I suffered birth trauma and subsequent perinatal post-traumatic stress disorder (PTSD) after the birth of my first daughter. My experience and the long battle to find support moved me to want to help others. So I created a website, Facebook and Twitter page called *Unfold Your Wings*. My desire was to raise awareness and offer hope and support for healing based on my personal journey to recovery. I have spent many years supporting women who have contacted me who have also suffered birth trauma.

My experiences led me to train as a Birth Buddy and to undertake training in perinatal mental health, trauma and all aspects of pregnancy, birth and parenting which has enabled me to support thousands of women and families in pregnancy, birth and beyond.

I am deeply passionate about improving maternity and maternal mental health services for women and their families. Today I'm privileged to work in the NHS caring for women, babies and families who have complex maternity journeys. I also use my experience and my knowledge from supporting families to help educate health professionals on the impact of trauma in birth, how to reduce birth trauma and improve support for families that are affected. I have been involved in many projects nationally to raise awareness of birth trauma, drive policy change and improve the care given in perinatal/maternal mental health and maternity services.

In 2018 I was honoured to win a THRIVE Mental Health Champion award for my volunteer work supporting families. I was also privileged to meet HRH the Princess of Wales for sharing my story as part of the 'Out of the blue' campaign with the charity Best Beginnings.

To describe me? Well, I'm quirky, creative, open-hearted and empathic. I don't mind being different and have never really followed the crowd. I'm passionate about things important to me. Sometimes a little insecure. I love flowers, trees, animals in fact all things nature, but especially butterflies as they have special meaning to me! I like nothing more than taking my camera to wonderful and interesting places and capturing life with all its magic. I love long summer days in my garden. The beach is one of my happy places too. Of course living in Wales the mountains, valleys and lakes are never far away.

I feel that my experiences in life especially my journey to healing have taught me so much. Sometimes life takes you down a path that may lead to places you never imagined. Sometimes things happen that change us forever, but even the bad I believe can be used for good.

I believe that things happen when we least expect them, and that surprise is part of the fabric of life too. We don't always know what awaits us in the rich tapestry of life, but when we are true to who we are, have companions that enrich our lives and we believe in ourselves, we can achieve anything. I hope I can inspire others to always be themselves and to see their inner strength, their self-worth and to know that they can overcome even the hardest of times to make a difference in the world.

1

WHERE IT ALL BEGAN

Six weeks too early my body was forced to give you up. I was failing you, failing to keep you safe and protected. My body was giving up, killing us both.

They took you from me, for only a second did I glimpse you. Your cry took ages to pierce the silence that hung heavy in the delivery room. The lights above me burned my eyes stinging with tears, as heavy footsteps rushed me down long corridors to the people that would save my life.

I couldn't remember what you looked like, only that you had wisps of golden hair. The mask filled my lungs to make me sleep and I was falling, falling into darkness, falling away from you.

When I woke a white figure stood before me and I felt a scream try to escape my throat. No this couldn't be true, an angel waiting for me, which meant I had left you without me, to never know me, for me to never hold you or tell you I loved you. Falling, I was falling again into the endless darkness, but I wasn't ready to let you go. Then light, voices, bleeping and pain but yes it meant life. A single tear fell, sliding down to dry cracked lips. Asking for water, asking for You. My body was too damaged I could not reach you, you felt a million miles away.

When I finally saw you in your glass box, a gift that was too priceless to behold. You curled your tiny hand around my finger and my heart I knew was no longer mine. You stole it, and, in that instant, I promised to never let you go.

So, I never left your side, a chair became my bed. All around me unkindness prevailed, but it would not keep me from you.

Moments became hours, hours to days, then weeks to months. Healing of body was slow, battered and bruised but slowly it faded. My mind was consumed its healing was far from approaching. Fear was now my daily companion. Your cry transported me back to that room, to the nights I was unable to be with you, to white figures seeking to claim me. You were mine now and I was a lioness protecting her young. I clutched you to my breast giving you the one thing I had, my milk. Everything around us became an enemy, nothing and no one would I let harm you. I wish I could hide you away from the world that was cold and bleak. To make sure that no pain would grace your door or turn your smiles away.

No one understood my secrets, nor did they seek to ask me why. Instead, I carried the pain and anguish all alone. Then I became blessed with your sister, to grow and bring into our world. Yet I believed that this time there would be no escape and I would certainly have to leave you both. Letters written with stained tear marks that told you both I loved you, lay among my nightwear, tiny baby clothes and nappies. Each day another day I got to love you both before I was ripped away. I tried to breathe you in, your scent and every detail. At night visions haunted me, falling again into the darkness, you both letting go of my hand.

Yet this time my body did not give out but instead protected where before it had not. With ease into the world came a daughter, with dark hair and with loud cries. Onto my chest, to hold and search, toes, fingers all so beautiful. I got to feel how it should be, to birth a baby and to both be free, to love and grow and be together moments you remember for all eternity.

Yet heal me it did not, for all I saw was you. My failure at everything you needed and the damage it had done. That I believed I had left you when you needed me most. That I couldn't protect you and of the things that we had lost.

Days became harder and fear became terror. I wanted to close my eyes and hope it all away. My love for you both was stronger than anything that could be thrown at me, but the trauma was tainting everything. Like a poison, it was seeping into our life. No one could offer me solace. No one understood. Alone and bereft it was the love of you both that kept me here.

So, began my search for help, my battle was raging, but I would not let it defeat me. The dark road ahead would be long and hard, but I knew that somehow, I would find the light again. For hope is stronger than fear, and my love for you both would conquer all. I knew that whatever it would take, I would find my way to heal *Beyond Birth Trauma.*

Unfolding my wings - beyond birth trauma

The birth of my first daughter changed my life, it changed me. As the lights passed above me as I was wheeled down the hospital corridor, I didn't think I would ever see my baby again, and I couldn't even remember what she looked like.

Anxiety, flashbacks and panic attacks became my life until I could barely function. For years I battled for help, passed around from service to service, wrong diagnosis after wrong diagnosis. Finally, I was seen and listened to by a clinical psychiatrist who finally saw and acknowledged what had happened to me and my trauma. She diagnosed me with Post Traumatic Stress Disorder (PTSD), caused by birth trauma and I cried with relief for 3 Days.

Yes, I had suffered birth trauma. It took me years to have what had happened to me at my daughter's birth acknowledged or even accepted. I was able to find someone who offered trauma counselling and this along with self-help helped me, as did finding others who had suffered birth trauma and reading about their experiences.

My road to healing though was long. I know how alone it can make you feel, so isolated and scared. Also, the impact it has on your life and how hard it can be to find help. As I began to recover I desperately wanted to change this, to help others, to raise awareness of birth trauma and perinatal PTSD. So I founded Unfold Your Wings a website and blog to offer hope for those who like me had suffered birth trauma and/or perinatal PTSD. This also in time led me to want to do more as I realised how many women were affected and yet how little it was talked about or its impact understood.

My birth trauma and subsequent struggle to get help for perinatal PTSD was a very painful and hard fight for many years. When I look back and reflect on my struggle to heal, I have realised, with time, that it has been a fight that has given to me, despite what it has taken away. It has given me the determination to try to help others who have also had birth trauma, reaching out to offer hope and support. It has driven me to try and improve the care given in maternity services, to try and prevent birth trauma in the first place.

I feel that what I experiencing has given me something special, a voice! That voice can speak out and sometimes shout loud about the need for things to change, both in the culture of pregnancy, birth and postnatal care but also the need for more support for perinatal mental health especially trauma on the maternity journey. I continue to always seek to use that voice to speak up for those who as yet are unable to speak out, to raise awareness of what birth trauma and perinatal PTSD are and to try to bring about change and improve, the care of women in birth.

It has been a privilege over the years to be able to voice my experience and the experiences of those I have supported by speaking at events and helping to train healthcare professionals to see how they can improve their practice, support families and reduce birth trauma. By also helping develop local and national policies and resources that help shape services for families. By doing so I hope that this has and will continue to mean that birth trauma is better understood.

I also know how important it is to have a safe place to share your story and be heard, to have your trauma acknowledged and how this helps you to heal. This too I have sought to offer others, a haven and solace in the darkest of times. A place where they can share what has happened to them and know that they are heard.

While birth trauma can cause so much pain, I believe in my heart that it is possible to find hope and life again beyond birth trauma. A dear friend when in the depths of my fight sent me a card that likened me to a butterfly. That while I had been in the dark cocoon of birth trauma with much struggle I was now breaking free and spreading my wings. This was so powerful to me and I have loved butterflies since! While they are fragile, they also have great strength and determination to break free and show their beauty. Like a butterfly I found ways to heal, to let my wings carry me to the light and do more than I ever thought possible. I hope that you too can find the light and healing again.

This book is my journey of healing from birth trauma. I hope the words it contains can give you hope and ways to help you on your journey. It contains what I have learned from my experience and how I healed beyond birth trauma. I hope that sharing my experience, how I sought to understand what had happened to me, and how I found peace may give you glimmers of light that you can use on your road to healing. While these are my experiences and what helped me, I know that healing is individual so I encourage you to search for what will help you to find recovery and healing.

The first chapters cover different aspects of **BEYOND**, the steps that helped me and I hope can help you as you walk your road to recovery. At the end of each chapter, I have included a reflection these are little exercises that can help you to reflect on what has been discussed in the chapter. Try each reflection and see what it brings to you personally. It doesn't matter how long it takes you to do it, minutes, days, weeks, or months. What matters is you are able to find time just for you, to spend time reflecting and see how it can help you to heal.

In the darkest of times, when you feel alone, knowing that someone else was struggling too but managed to find their way into the light can be a source of strength and solace.

So, come with me, take my hand, open your heart and let us together explore healing *Beyond Birth Trauma.*

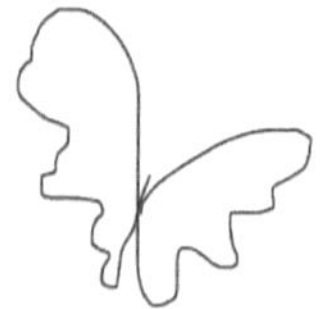

POEM

Instead of you against my chest,
they took you away, I tried my best.

The lights above hurt my eyes,
no one could hear my inner cries.

Their last words fill my ears,
quick, or else we lose her here.

Was I alive, I couldn't tell.
Was this an angel to bid my farewell?

In HDU strange smells, and sounds,
doctors coming, going doing their rounds.

Many days without you near,
filling me with doubt and fear.

Then your tiny face, a touch of your hand,
in a plastic box, this is not what I planned.

On the ward instead of love and care,
cruel words, sadly compassion was nowhere.

Physical scars slowly healed,
but emotionally I had no shield.

PTSD became my chalice,
filling my days and nights with malice.

Mothers, babies and families matter,
a difficult birth can leave their dreams shattered.

2

WHAT IS BIRTH TRAUMA?

**"Birth trauma is in the eye of the beholder."
Cheryl Beck**

Birth can be a wondrous time for families. The bringing of a new life into the arms of its parents. A time to rejoice, build memories and look forward to the new road of parenthood. For many, this is a happy time, full of excitement and joy. A time when families are born and parents are made.

However this isn't always the case, sadly for some families, birth is instead a time of anxiety, stress and anguish. The birth of their baby instead of being a positive experience has been so difficult they are left feeling huge distress, even traumatised. When birth has been a traumatic time the impact is overwhelming feelings that are hard to understand, and overshadow what they feel should be a happy and joyous time. It can leave new parents feeling disappointed, frustrated and even angry at their birth experience and the early days and weeks with their new baby.

So why can birth be traumatic? Well, when it comes to pregnancy and birth each woman's* experience is unique to her. How she feels about her birth experience is important and it is also true that what one woman may find traumatic, another may not. Birth is as individual as the person, and this applies also to the impact of birth trauma.

There can be many reasons a woman feels her birth was traumatic. It may be that it was a frightening event that made her feel overwhelmed and out of control. It may have been an emergency situation where her life and/or that of her baby was at risk, many women voiced that they believed that they were dying or they were losing their baby.

Maybe labour was very lengthy and/or very painful causing huge distress or for some women, it can be the opposite and instead, their birth was very fast and intense.

Sometimes birth may have complications that mean medical interventions are needed, such as induction, caesarean section, episiotomy, assisted delivery or other medical procedures. Again this can cause distress, especially in an emergency situation.

Some babies may be born early or sick and require care in a neonatal unit which again can bring great distress to parents, with some spending many weeks or months being cared for in a neonatal unit.

It can also be that birth was traumatic not because negative things happened, but instead because there was a loss of positive things such as a much-wanted birth experience, whatever that may look like for that woman or family.

Sadly too, despite all the advances in medical care, birth can result in damage or injury to a mother and/or her baby. This can mean life-changing circumstances for a family both in terms of recovery, where this is possible, or the acceptance of long-term health or medical conditions to the woman or her baby that may have resulted from a difficult birth.

Of course, we know that for some families birth can mean the loss of their baby, which is devastating and traumatic for a whole family.

What else can cause women to feel traumatised? It can be a woman may feel a loss of control, dignity and privacy. There may have been a lack of information given about her care or procedures that were advised. A woman may feel she wasn't listened to in her birth and her choices not respected, or even overlooked and ignored. She may feel she had medical procedures done to her without her consent or proper explanation. That she had no choices offered around her care or that the choices made were not informed choices, even that she was coerced into a procedure or situation that she did not want.

There may be situations where her culture, beliefs or emotional needs were not understood or respected. Some may experience trauma due to health, social and economic inequalities. Others may have found that they didn't receive the support they needed in relation to their race, gender or sexual orientation. Or that a previous history of trauma or mental health issues was not considered.

For some on paper, their birth may have looked 'perfect' and yet for reasons very personal to them, they may have found it deeply traumatic. This can be especially challenging and many have voiced that have felt unable to say they how deeply they have been affected.

Often women will say it was the language used that caused them trauma which was unkind, cruel or damaging. Others voice that their care was without compassion or empathy or in some cases they felt neglected and abandoned.

For some women, they find their pregnancy or birth experience re-triggers or can add to, previous trauma such as rape, domestic or childhood abuse. Often finding that this wasn't something they could disclose to those over their care, they have tried to manage the impact of their traumas. Some as a result labelled difficult, hard to engage with and challenging. Even when able to reveal previous trauma many have found that the care offered wasn't trauma-informed, instead failing to take into account their needs and they were left reeling in the aftermath.

It's not just the birth itself but women can find that a difficult pregnancy contributed to feeling traumatised and this was the source of their birth trauma. This can be greatly overlooked and women can feel that their concerns and anxieties are often dismissed or minimised. Especially can this be so if women have had multiple miscarriages or the difficult journey of fertility treatment. Often the narrative is that the focus should now be on this pregnancy and can discount the long journey already taken, the emotional impact and the need to feel emotionally safe this time.

It may be that the pregnancy and birth were in themselves positive but then they felt traumatised by poor postnatal care, lack of infant feeding support, complications in the postnatal period or the sudden onset or re-triggering of mental health issues. Families are often left feeling abandoned, and alone trying to manage difficult challenges at such a vulnerable time as they begin their journey as parents.

Whatever the reasons, trauma from birth is real and this must be acknowledged and understood. Without this, recovery is hard and finding the right support to heal, is almost impossible.

The aftermath of birth trauma

So what is the aftermath when birth is traumatic? One of the biggest is how birth trauma impacts relationships.

Women who feel traumatised from their birth often feel isolated and alone with feelings they struggle to share after all the birth of a baby should be a celebrated time and admitting that this isn't the case has instead left them feeling traumatised, can be hard to understand, and admit.

Family and friends and sometimes even partners may not understand why a woman feels traumatised. This can leave her feeling guilty or somehow weak for not being able to 'cope' with her birth experience. She may believe that she should be able to just 'get over' her birth experience and move on. This can damage relationships with partners, family members and friends as a woman feels no one understands her feelings and the impact on her. She may as a result feel silenced, and this can cause her to withdraw from those who love her, even breaking trust in relationships. Being unable to say how deeply she has been affected by her experience to anyone can also mean a delay in receiving much-needed help and support.

Sex within a relationship may also be affected as a woman may fear further pregnancies or even just the act of physical intimacy itself. This can lead to feelings of guilt and put immense stress on relationships, even the breakdown of relationships as a couple tries to navigate the impact birth trauma has had on them. Even just being affectionate can be hard as she struggles to deal with the flood of emotions she may be feeling, causing her to withdraw and isolate herself from her partner, family and friends. Any physical damage from the birth will impact the intimate side of relationships. Recovery can be long and a woman's body can feel different which can affect her body image and self-confidence. When a mind is dealing with the aftermath of birth trauma, the body feels it too.

Women are often told, *at least you are okay now, or you have a healthy baby,* while often said out of well-meaning motives it can leave them feeling like their experience is dismissed or somehow not really that bad. However, a healthy baby isn't all that matters. Women too need to be well both physically and emotionally.

What about the relationship with her baby? A mother and her baby are a dyad, each connected to the other. What affects one affects the other. Many women who suffer birth trauma find their relationship with their baby is affected too. They may struggle to bond with their babies causing huge guilt. Some even find their baby a constant trigger or reminder of the birth and that they didn't feel the expected deep connection straight away, or they blame the birth of their baby for all the trauma that they now feel.

After a traumatic birth some women are so unwell they have not been able to hold or care for their new baby. This greatly impacts those first moments, hours, days and weeks with their newborn. Many will struggle with great guilt and grief due to this, that they didn't get to be with their baby during those early hours and days.

Others may become overly anxious over their baby's health and well-being and constantly worry about every aspect of caring for their baby. They may live in perpetual fear of harm coming to their baby, or experience separation anxiety and struggle to allow anyone else to help with caring for their baby. Intrusive thoughts may happen about their baby which can be frightening and again cause great distress. They may constantly fear they are not a good mother and seek reassurance from those around them.

For a woman who has lost a baby or whose baby has been injured during birth, there may be the experience of overwhelming guilt. She may feel like it is her fault, that she somehow failed her baby or that she should somehow have prevented it. That maybe something she did or didn't do has meant harm to her baby. This adds to the trauma and profound loss that is already painful and devastating. This can lead to women replaying the events of birth over and over seeking to find answers to what could have changed the outcome. The result can be a downward spiral of anguish, pain, guilt and self-blame.

Another aspect that can be affected is a woman may feel unable to attend healthcare appointments or have further medical tests or treatments. This can especially be so if poor care has contributed to a traumatic birth, as trust is then broken with healthcare professionals and so accessing support for anything of a medical nature can be difficult. If there is physical trauma being able to attend appointments such as smear tests can be a huge source of stress and cause a re-triggering of their experience of birth. So too can returning to the place of birth trauma, such as the hospital where she gave birth. This may be needed to attend appointments either for herself or her baby, however, this can re-trigger painful memories and emotions. As a result, women may avoid getting the care they need as they feel unable to cope with the emotional and physical responses that result.

It is therefore an understatement to say that birth trauma profoundly impacts women and families. When a traumatic birth happens it can leave devastation in its wake.

What happens when birth trauma is overlooked or misunderstood? It can result in being wrongly diagnosed, often as other conditions such as postnatal depression.

Women report they are rarely asked how they feel about their birth experience and how it has impacted them emotionally. In the postnatal period, they may feel very anxious or low in mood yet this may not be linked by those around them in any way to the birth. This can mean the right support isn't offered for the reason they are actually struggling, which is due to a difficult pregnancy or birth experience.

For others, it may be that they disassociate from everything and everyone around them in order to cope with their birth experience and its aftermath, including their baby. Again this may not be seen in the context of the birth experience by those caring for families and so the right support is not offered. Instead, women can be labelled as detached from their babies, not coping or bonding, without seeing the trauma behind it.

Perinatal PTSD

For some so severe is their trauma it can lead to developing Post Traumatic Stress Disorder (PTSD). It is estimated that, in the UK alone, up to 30.000 women a year find some part of their birth traumatic**. Most will overcome this with the right support. However, research suggests that about 4-5 % of women develop Post-Traumatic Stress Disorder (PTSD) from their traumatic birth, which will need additional specialist professional mental health support and treatment. This is estimated because this doesn't include those who do not speak out about their suffering, who are not acknowledged as having had a traumatic birth, or who are misdiagnosed. This also does not include partners, healthcare professionals or birth workers who also may suffer birth trauma.

What is Post-Traumatic Stress Disorder (PTSD)? Simply it is the clinical term for experiencing normal reactions to a traumatic, distressing experience or event. It can occur after a person experiences or witnesses something that was, or they perceive to have been, life-threatening. Many have heard of this concerning soldiers returning from war, or after experiencing a life-threatening event such as a natural disaster, but we often do not relate it to the birth of a baby. Yet birth-related PTSD is very real and affects many families.

Signs of perinatal PTSD include feelings of intense fear, helplessness and/or terror. Re-experiencing the events of the birth by recurrent intrusive memories, flashbacks and/or nightmares.

Other signs are feeling distressed, anxious or panicked when exposed to something which reminds them of the birth. This then can result in avoidance of anything that is a reminder of pregnancy or birth. This can include talking about it, going to or near the place where their birth happened such as hospitals, or the people that may have been involved in the trauma, like doctors, or other healthcare professionals. It can even be television programs or books that show or mention birth. Some women also struggle when any of their friends or family may be pregnant or have just given birth, and they may avoid contact with them or attendance at social events associated with pregnancy or birth.

Bad memories or flashbacks of the birth can lead to difficulties with sleeping or concentrating and other daily activities such as eating, drinking or caring for their needs. Women may also feel angry, irritable and be hyper-vigilant or jumpy, and easily startled. Some may suffer panic attacks, depression or/and anxiety or other mental health conditions.

Others may feel detached, and alone and have a sense that something bad may happen to them or their loved ones at any time. Dissociation can occur, a disconnection between their thoughts, memories, feelings, actions, or sense of who they are. This can involve 'losing touch' with awareness of one's immediate surroundings and can happen during flashbacks where they may be taken back to images of the event. All this can be frightening and cause great distress especially while trying to care for a new baby.

It is important to understand that PTSD is beyond the person's control. It is the mind's way of trying to make sense of an extremely traumatic experience and is not a sign of an individual's weakness or inability to cope. They cannot just 'get over it' or 'pull themselves together' or 'move on'. Rather they need help and support to process not only what has happened to them, but also the feelings surrounding it, and how it has affected the way they now think and perceive the world. Trauma is a nervous system that is stuck in 'threat', unable to switch off the body's reactions. Things that previously may have gone unnoticed or not a source of distress can now induce fear and very real physical sensations. We can understand then why this would be especially challenging in the postnatal period with a new baby to care for.

There are various treatments for perinatal PTSD that are effective and it is important that women are able to reach out for help and access them. They can speak to their healthcare providers such as a Midwife, Health Visitor or GP about how they are feeling who can then support them in getting help. Some areas allow for self-referral to mental health services for assessment and therapies. Early intervention is important, as is accessing the right support. It can be scary asking for help and many will voice they worry about how they will be viewed but taking that first step will mean they can receive the support they need to recover before the roots of trauma take a firm hold.

PTSD is real and its effects can be devastating. Sufferers often feel alone and isolated like they are in a cocoon of darkness. However, there are treatments and therapies that work and families need to know that it is possible to recover with the right help.

It is also important that those caring for families during pregnancy, birth and the postnatal period are aware of the signs of birth trauma and perinatal PTSD and know how to help families and support them in finding the right help.

In conclusion, birth trauma is real, it is important that if a woman is struggling emotionally or physically following the birth of her baby, she is asked about her maternity journey including her birth experience and given time to talk about her feelings, as well as offered and helped to access any support she may need.

Healing from birth trauma is possible with the right help and support, but the first step is the awareness that it exists and the trauma acknowledged. It is wrong to think that a difficult birth can just be forgotten or wished away. Time does not wipe away the pain as many are told, the reality is that when birth trauma is not seen and validated, but instead ignored, it can be carried by a woman her entire life.

If you have read this chapter and feel that you may have birth trauma or perinatal PTSD reach out for help. Speak to those around you and tell them how you feel. Seek out the right services that can offer you the therapies to heal and recover. It will be hard but the right thing for you and your family.

After the right diagnosis and support I finally was able to start my road to healing beyond birth trauma, so join me as we explore together what helped me along the way.

*While I refer to women or use the pronouns she/her throughout the book, I acknowledge that not all individuals will identify as such. Also, partners, healthcare professionals and birth workers may be the ones who are suffering and affected by birth trauma.

** Figures from The Birth Trauma Association

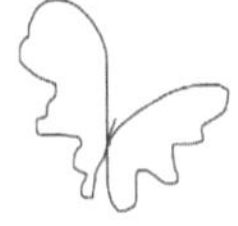

3

HEALING COMES FROM WITH-IN

"She took her broken pieces and made them into wings."

**"I never believed that healing was possible for me,
but then with the right support, I was able to see I
deserved to find peace again."**
Kirsty

Healing after birth trauma is possible, but it will be as individual to each person as the experience itself. I always think of it as a road laid out before us that leads to a new destination. Each journey will be different, and so will the time needed. The road may be long, or it may be short. Some will process their experience and feelings quickly, for others healing may take many months, even years.

It doesn't matter how long you need on your road, how you travel, or who is with you along the way. It also doesn't matter what others think about your journey. What does matter is that the road to healing is yours to start, and while this journey will not be straight or easy, instead hard and with some obstacles to overcome, you can travel it, and eventually reach your destination.

The road to healing is complex. Sometimes you may need to stop and rest as you walk your road to healing, this is ok as it will allow you to glance behind and see how far you have already come. Sometimes you may look ahead and doubt you can carry on because the way doesn't seem clear or you may fear what lies ahead, yet this will give you space to see what you need to keep moving on your journey. There may be times when the road feels just too hard, and you will need others to help you. This is when they will take your hand gently urging you on, or maybe they will carry you for a while until you're strong enough to take some steps on your own again. Others may just sit with you as you rest and help you to decide where to go next.

Frustration also may walk with you for a while as you desperately wish to jump to the end of the journey, to be at that final destination, free from the pain and turmoil that seems to be your daily companion. However, there are no shortcuts I wish there were. Your road must be walked, but you can do it with tiny steps that get you there, at the pace that is right for you.

So, the question is what does healing beyond birth trauma mean to you? I'm guessing that if you're reading this book you're looking for the answer just like I was. I have been there, desperate to heal but not knowing where to turn. In the beginning, I didn't even know what healing was for me. Healing means different things to different people and finding your healing is a personal quest. Healing is whatever that means for you, there is no wrong or right answer.

In the depth of my struggle with birth trauma and the darkness it cast that invaded my life, the search for 'my cure' became an endless battle. I was desperate, and the need to fix myself consumed my thoughts and my days. I would have tried anything. I researched until my eyes hurt as much as my mind. A never-ending quest to banish the monster that walked with me daily. Healing became everything. I had been changed and all I wanted was to be me again, to find the life that I had before. I believed that there would be some magical formula that would transform me, remove the trauma and make everything ok.

Medication, tapping, challenging my thoughts, hypnosis, positive thinking and other techniques all became part of my repertoire. A juggling act of hope that something would work. Of the many therapists I saw, few offered any answers. At the start, I would be told they could cure me, that this would be my healing. I would often have worksheets thrust at me, things to do over and over, or boxes and diagrams to fill out. Yet when I didn't improve, when my cure didn't happen, frustration would result from the therapist and myself. I would be told that the failure lay with me. 'I wasn't trying hard enough', 'I wasn't practising enough' or 'I wasn't doing it', (whatever 'it' was) correctly.

Others made me believe that I was the problem. I was told to move on, to try to forget my trauma, to just get over it. I was told I was missing out on life, and to pull myself together. One therapist even said to me that I liked suffering, that I got some form of pleasure from it and that I was causing it all myself.

So, the darkness grew deeper. I became more lost. Guilt consumed me, I felt defective and to blame for all the hurt I believed I was incurring on myself and also so I believed, those I loved. Healing seemed impossible for me. An unreachable destination of which I had no idea how I was going to get there.

Of course, the main reason was because then I didn't know what the cause of my pain was. I had never heard of birth trauma, didn't know that it even existed. All I knew was that I was hurting and that the person I had been, was gone. The girl who was happy, outgoing and full of life was now ripped away and instead, what was left was someone broken and in pain. Fear was my daily companion and I felt so very alone. No one seemed to understand, and I had become accustomed to the frowns and quizzical looks that adorned the faces of those to whom I tried to bare my soul. I would be told that I should enjoy my baby and try to embrace life and be grateful but it felt impossible to me and I didn't understand why.

The turning point for me came when I was given a safe space to talk about my birth experience. When instead of dismissal, I was listened to. It wasn't in a therapist's office but in a room of women where our birth stories mattered. For the first time, empathy and love were held out to me, nothing more. This was for me what I needed most. That safe space and unconditional acceptance allowed for a tiny glimmer of light. No one told me that I needed to get over what had happened, instead, they just listened and let me tell my story, purging my soul of all that I had been carrying. With this acceptance that my birth experience had impacted me so deeply, I was able to start my road to healing.

I knew that I needed the right support, support that allowed me to see a way to healing but this was so hard to find. By accident, I found a therapist who had been through trauma herself and knew it intimately. No worksheets were offered, and no quick cures were promised, instead, I was given my voice, in a quiet room where I could speak from my heart, where I could cry and lament the pain that I had held in for so long. My trauma was finally acknowledged, in every raw, distressing detail. I was able to grieve it all, the pain, the loss, the things it had taken from me. I was able to explore what I had previously been denied, that the way I was feeling was because the birth of my daughter instead of being a wonderful joyous event, had damaged me physically and mentally. That I wasn't to blame, I wasn't causing it, I wasn't defective or not trying hard enough. No, I had been traumatised and then left to deal with it all on my own while also trying to care for my new baby. I began to understand my feelings, my emotions, what trauma was and why I was struggling. It was profound in so many ways.

As time passed, I realised I didn't need a cure. What I needed was compassion and understanding. I needed acknowledgement of what I had been through. I needed a listening kind heart and a safe space. What I also needed was to know that how I felt mattered, and that my experience was important. That I mattered. This was the start of my healing journey.

I also began to realise something else. While healing could be done with the help of others, ultimately it came from within me. Others could guide me, support me and give me the space I needed, but the rest came from understanding my trauma, how I felt about it and then finding ways to deal with my trauma. There was no magic cure, no secret way to fix me. Instead, I needed to see that while I was changed, I was still me. Instead of looking to others to cure me, I realised that healing lay with me.

Healing came from accepting the changes, understanding them and growing from them. This we will look at later in the book and at this point that may feel impossible for you. Healing came from knowing I wasn't defective but hurt, a victim who needed time to recover. It still amazes me that birth trauma seems to be the only trauma where recovery is overlooked. I remember a friend who not long after I had my daughter was in a car accident where she broke her leg. She was inundated with cards, flowers, offers of homemade food and people to do her shopping, an understanding of the pain she was in physically and emotionally. That understanding is important after birth trauma too.

I have lost count of the times I've seen new mums attempting to carry on and 'get back to normal' despite the most traumatic of births, usually with their trauma left unacknowledged. Sadly, this is an issue that society has missed to the detriment of families everywhere, the result being many struggling with the impact of birth trauma.

Healing also came from instead of trying to fix what I saw as something wrong with me, to being able to see that what I actually needed was to be kind to myself. For so long I had been berating myself for not being ok, for believing I was weak and for not 'coping'. I needed to learn to let go of what I felt I should be, to understand that my trauma needed time to heal and also to see how far I had already come on my journey. That while I had been touched by trauma, and that it had changed me and my life beyond all recognition, I was ready to embrace it and find my way to healing. I also needed to see that it didn't have to define me or my life from that point on.

So, too with you. Your trauma cannot be undone, and this is heartbreaking to say. What can be undone is the impact that it is having on you, both emotionally and physically. Healing is right there within you. I know you may not know it, you may even not believe it and that's ok right now. I didn't believe it either and it has taken a long journey to find out that it is true. I can only say that you will find your healing, whatever that looks like for you.

Bad Days Are Part of Your Journey

The road to healing however isn't easy. Some days will be hard. Some days will be dark. Some days you will want to give up and think you can't go on. It is easy to allow the bad days to knock you off the road to healing and make you believe that you're just not getting anywhere.

If you were to ask me, I would say that I am healed. I am healed from the trauma that was my daughter's birth, which changed me and my life. However, if you asked me, does this mean that I no longer have bad days, my answer would be, no.

There are still days where I struggle, where my anxiety plagues me, and I want to run and hide from the world. I still have days filled with self-doubt, where I am my worst critic and guilt creeps in. I still have days where difficult memories return. Sometimes those bad days become bad patches, lasting longer than I would like, making me twitchy and nervous.

Sadly, for a long time, I berated myself for the bad days. After all, I believed that I had to be perfect for my family, I had to be cured and back to the old me. I would view the bad days as a failure, that I had lost my way again and then everything else would become defined by that bad day. As the dark cloud descended, my memory would become selective. I would forget all the positive days, all the things I had achieved and could do. I would lose sight of my journey and how far I had travelled on my road to recovery. Instead, I would question if I was making any progress at all and so the spiral in my thoughts would start and I would feel like I was at the bottom of a deep hole.

What can a bad day look like? Sometimes it's having to cancel something you have planned or having to let someone down. Sometimes it is forgetting to take needed rest or practice self-care. Other times it is struggling to get through the day, be it at work or caring for your family. On some bad days, you will struggle to cope with being a parent as well as you would like to, your patience on a shoestring, that crushed cornflake in the carpet being the final straw. On other bad days, you may barely function at all, the pain and anguish leaving you exhausted and emotionally low. Each bad day can be different with varying emotions, such as sadness, anger or guilt. I'm sure you could add many more to this list and your bad days may look very different to mine. Not all bad days may be seen either, you may cover them well, masquerading your true feelings as you try to carry on.

Part of healing is accepting that this means bad days will visit you. Your bad days whether on their own or ones that stretch into weeks are part of your journey too. As you learn to accept them, they will lose the hold they have on you, because you know that they will eventually pass. You will be able to see that they do not mean you are not healing, in fact, the opposite, they show you are healing, walking that road, doing all you can to keep going. Gradually those days will become less and there will be many more good days, than bad.

When I reflected on my bad days, I often saw that they were trying to tell me something. Sometimes they were telling me I had done too much, and that I needed to stop, take care of myself and rest. Other times I was expecting too much of myself, that I had lost healthy boundaries and I needed reminding that I didn't need to be perfect. They also allowed me to seek where I was placing my attention and if I was neglecting myself again. It's so easy to place ourselves at the bottom of the pile with everything and everyone else taking priority, especially with a family to care for. We are quick to forget that we matter too and that in order to care for others we must first care for ourselves.

My bad days reminded me too that I am a survivor of trauma and as such my journey to healing would be ongoing. I needed my bad days to help me see the good, to help me see that I was getting there, no matter how long it took. They reminded me that I was stronger than I realised, even on the days that I felt weak, that I had gotten through them before and would do so again.

Bad days also help you to stop and take stock of what you need to heal. They allow you to re-assess what is or isn't working.

Sometimes bad days come because they are part of you working through your experience or therapy you are undertaking. Triggers and memories will also come to visit you at times and these too can lead to bad days.

Anniversaries and birthdays can be especially hard days as they can cause traumatic memories to resurface and cause you to feel guilty for finding it hard to celebrate them as 'happy times.' This is something we will look at later on in the book.

There are two things you can do to prevent bad days from stopping you in your tracks. First, allow the bad days to be a time of reflection. Stop, turn around and see how far you have come. Think about how much you have accomplished and how strong you are. On a bad day, it may be all you can do to get out of bed and survive the day. See this as the achievement it is! Everyone has bad days no matter who they are. Now look at you. Look at what you have been through. Look at the progress you are making. Look at those around you and how much they love and need you. See the road behind you winding away into the distance, it is gone, you're not going that way anymore, instead, see clearly the road ahead and the strength you possess. Let this inspire you to carry on one step at a time.

Second. Do what you need to do to get through the bad day. Maybe it means you need to rest. Maybe you need to distract yourself, maybe you need to cry and grieve or reach out for support. Maybe you need to get out of the house and walk off some of the pain or talk to a valued and trusted friend. Finding healthy ways to support you is so important. Also, remember no matter how dark the day is there will be better days, you have got through worse days than this and you will do it again. You have fought to get this far. Just as the bad day appeared, so it will pass. All you need to do is manage your bad day using the things that help you. Do not resist them as this can in turn only seek to emphasise them but let them reside a while until you can move on again. I guarantee you it will pass and you will carry on your road to healing.

Bad days do not mean you are failing.
Bad days do not mean you are not making progress.
Bad days do not mean you are not healing.

Bad days are just that, a bad day, and tomorrow you will lift up your head, and start the fight again. Reach out to those who can support you while you let the bad day pass. Take their hand and let them help. Or if you need to rest for a while, let them rest with you, there by your side. There is so much comfort to be found in the arms of those who know your journey.

Your bad days are just like stones on the road, that have caused you to stumble. Yet each time they do, pick yourself up and carry on. Do not let it cause you to doubt your journey because you have travelled so very far. Healing isn't just your destination; healing is your whole journey. Healing means carrying on, allowing the days that are hard to come and reside with you for a while until they pass again. Healing means listening to what they are telling you and making sure you are caring for yourself. Yes, healing doesn't mean you no longer have bad days. I promise you that before long you will find those bad days are less and less and instead you will have many more good days that support your healing journey.

Finding the right support

After a traumatic birth finding the right support is important. This can be hard because it is often when you feel at your most vulnerable that you will need to ask for help. It can be difficult to know what will help you on your road to healing.

If you are struggling do not suffer in silence. Speak to someone, a partner, family or a trusted friend. Tell them you are struggling and ask them to help you. This may be in practical ways such as help with daily tasks. It may be emotionally by providing that safe space you need to talk and pour out your heart. Communicating what you need is important as they may not understand how your birth has impacted you. You can also ask loved ones to advocate for you when you are struggling, such as coming with you to therapy appointments or even making the appointment for you.

You can also approach your Midwife, Health Visitor, GP or local Mental Health Service (UK). In some areas, you can self-refer for support, be it counselling or other therapy. This can be especially hard to do if trust in healthcare services or professionals has been broken by perhaps poor care. This is where your family can support you to liaise with those who can offer help to get the support you need. It is also important, to be honest with services and healthcare professionals about what you have been through, how it has impacted you and that you are finding it hard to build again the trust that has been broken.

After a difficult birth, you may also have many questions about what happened. It is usually possible to make an appointment at the hospital where you gave birth to review the medical notes of your birth to discuss exactly what happened and why. This is often called a 'birth debrief'. Some hospitals offer 'birth reflection' sessions for you to talk about your birth, ask any questions you may have and then feedback on your concerns. Usually, this is offered by a Midwife or a Consultant Doctor who may have been at your birth. Debriefs or birth reflections are usually offered when you are at least six weeks postpartum but can be accessed at any time, even years after your birth experience.

There is a lot of discussion around how helpful a debrief or a birth reflection session may be and it will depend on how it is conducted and by whom. A debrief can help to fill in any blanks you may have about your birth experience or allow you to ask any questions about your care or any interventions.

If you decide to have a debrief be aware that this is often about the medical aspect of your birth and not always the emotional. Support before and after can make a huge difference, especially being able to talk about what you may have learned in your debrief. Talk with those who are offering the debrief about what it will entail and take someone with you such as a partner or family member/ friend who can offer support. It is a good idea to make a list of the things you would like to ask or the concerns you may have about what happened.

Some hospitals use debriefs to draw on issues that families are raising to help improve the care given in maternity. Be honest and open about how you are feeling and have been impacted by your experience. This way those who conduct your debrief inform services of the points you raise to try and make changes.

I've attended many debriefs over the years with families and on the whole, they have been beneficial and helped with processing the events. I have however also heard from many women for whom this hasn't been the case. Some caution is therefore needed around awareness of protecting your emotional well-being and understanding that a debrief may help support you to heal but may also not give you all the answers you hoped for.

What kind of support may you be offered to help you after birth trauma?

Therapies that may be offered for birth trauma can be varied. It may include counselling, Eye Movement Desensitisation and Reprocessing (EMDR), Cognitive Behavioural Therapy (CBT) and medication. I do not recommend any particular one as from personal experience and from supporting many individuals, finding the right therapy takes time and is different for everyone.

Do your research and find what works for you. Remember your journey of healing is unique to you and as such it means experimenting with various therapies to find the right match to meet your needs.

Cognitive behavioural therapy (CBT) is often offered to help with coping after trauma. It supports you to challenge unhelpful thoughts and worries and think about them differently. This can be helpful after a traumatic birth to help with how you may be thinking about your world after your experience. CBT helps you to challenge thoughts that are causing you anxiety or distress. It can give you coping strategies for distressing thoughts or memories. CBT sessions are usually offered over around 6-8 weeks but can be offered for longer.

Counselling can also be of benefit to help process and come to terms with trauma from a difficult birth. Talking with someone about your experience can offer a release and time to reflect on how you have been affected. This is often where the safe space I mentioned earlier is possible.

Feeling heard and not judged, provides much in the way of healing. I personally found trauma counselling to be really helpful and definitely supported me as I navigated my recovery.

Eye Movement Desensitisation and Reprocessing (EMDR) is a treatment especially used for those who have experienced trauma. During EMDR therapy sessions, you recall traumatic or triggering experiences while a therapist directs your eye movements. EMDR is thought to be effective because recalling traumatic events is often less upsetting when your attention is diverted. This allows you to be exposed to the memories without having a strong psychological response. Over time, this technique is believed to lessen the impact that the memories or thoughts have on you. It allows for the processing of trauma without having to talk about it or relive it. It can help a traumatic experience become a coherent event in the past, instead of overwhelming images, sensations, and emotions in the present. I have heard many report that they have found EMDR to be helpful with the distressing memories of their birth, again it is good to find what works for you.

Mindfulness is another approach that can help you to become aware of your thoughts and feelings to see how they are limiting to you. It helps you to remain in the present with an awareness of your past experiences and how they are affecting you now. It can provide coping strategies for feelings of anxiety or overwhelm. It can be especially helpful in later healing to allow our minds to rest and relax. Many view mindfulness as meditation or breathing exercises, however, mindfulness can be many things including a refreshing walk on a bright, sunny day.

Medication will sometimes be offered/prescribed which can help lessen the emotional symptoms of birth trauma such as anxiety and provide much-needed respite to aid recovery. Medication can provide needed support to help you manage the often-distressing impact of trauma. It is important that you discuss your needs with your doctor including any side effects that you may experience. While medication can help lessen the symptoms of trauma it is good to also combine this with a therapy that helps with the processing of your experience. If you are breastfeeding talk to your healthcare provider as there are safe medications you can take while continuing to feed your baby.

When seeking support for birth trauma it can be a minefield knowing who to trust. False promises, unrealistic guarantees and experimental therapies can lead to damage. Also, remember that if any treatments are as effective as they claim there will be research to back this up. Ideally, any therapist you seek should have been through the therapy that they themselves offer. It is perfectly okay and reasonable to ask about their training and if they have personally benefited from the therapy they are offering you.

So, when looking at therapy ask, what are the results that are being promised? Is there a promise of a cure or a quick result? Is what is being promised realistic? Is the therapy evidence-based? Is the therapy right for you and your situation? Do you feel there is some improvement as the therapy progresses?

Remember also that everyone is an individual, with unique experiences, personalities and needs. Not all therapies will work for everyone. This doesn't mean that there is anything wrong with you as a person, only that the particular treatment wasn't right. Finding what does work can take time. It took me a long time to find what worked for me.

Any therapist who insists that their therapy is the only

one that will work for you is only interested in their own benefits and not in truly helping you to heal. Therapy should be flexible, and you should always be part of all your care planning.

What about the person offering the therapy? How do they make you feel? Does the person you are being supported by make you feel safe? Do you feel they are looking at you as an individual with your own history and needs, without judgement? Do you sense a genuine wish to help you or are you just another client, another list of symptoms or diagnosis? Are they open to learning from you too? Do you get the sense they understand your trauma and how it is affecting you? Important questions for you to personally consider. Sadly, I came across many therapists who only made my struggle worse often due to not understanding the impact of trauma especially in relation to birth. I learned the hard way that not everyone who promises to help you will do just that!

So too with this book, it isn't to replace the therapy that you need, rather it is to provide ideas that I found helpful as I healed that you can try. There will be parts of it that you will find helpful and maybe some not so. It is important that you seek out and access the right help for you to recover. Healing is your personal journey but I want you to know that your healing lies within you, it's just about finding it. I hope that this book will be with you along the way, like a companion. That it will give you hope and help you to know that while recovery from birth trauma may be a long and difficult journey, it is possible. I hope that by sharing my journey with you and what helped me, you too can find your way along the road to healing.

Finding local support groups or support groups on social media (such as the Birth Trauma Association) can also support your road to healing too. Peer support from those who have had similar experiences can help you feel less alone and allow for the sharing of things that can help you as you heal.

Healing is possible.

Healing doesn't mean that the pain never existed. It doesn't mean you forget. Healing instead means you see your experience in a new way, as something that while is part of you, that from time to time will still bring you pangs of pain, it is no longer in control of you. Healing means taking the strength that lies within you and letting it grow, like a seedling that though buried in the dark pushes forth to reach the light. With each step, with each small victory, your strength and steps to healing increase.

Healing is yours and yours alone. There is no time scale and no expectations. It is a journey that you can choose to take. Everyone will heal differently, and everyone's meaning of healing will be different. Yet it is possible to heal in the way that is right for you. Remember healing is as much about recovery as it is about remembering how you survived what hurt you. Remember too that healing doesn't mean you forget what you have been through. Healing means that while birth trauma is what happened to you, it's not who you are. You have been touched by birth trauma, you may not be the same person you once were, your life may have been changed forever and while you cannot wipe away all that you have suffered, you can find your way to heal beyond birth trauma. This will mean you will find ways to cope with, accept and adapt, to the changes it has made to you and your life.

Healing is possible, it is deep within you. So, find those buried seeds of hope, feed, nurture and help them grow. Let others, guide and support you. Most of all believe, that you can do this. Healing is your journey. Every day rejoice at how far you have come and cherish every little step. Whatever your journey to healing never give up, keep going, and don't let the bad days push you off the road or self-doubt cause you to stumble, keeping you from moving ahead.

While the road is scary and unchartered, remember you are not alone. Around you are the voices, strength and support of everyone who loves you, and those who like you, are walking their road to healing too.

Yes, it is possible to heal. It is possible to heal beyond birth trauma.

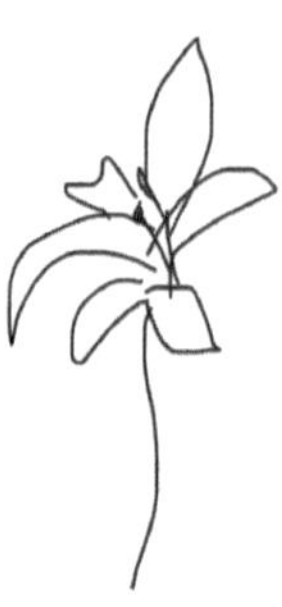

A reflection for you.

Take some time to think about what healing means to you. Do you just want to feel better, or do you want life to be better? Do you feel open to starting your journey to healing and what does this mean for you? What does the road ahead look like?

On a piece of paper draw a road leading off into the horizon. See yourself on the road. Draw on the horizon something that represents a healed you.

Then write on your road the things that healing means to you.

- Your feelings, hopes, and wishes for a healed you.
- What are your hopes, fears and perceived obstacles to healing?
- Who/what can help you navigate the road to healing?
- Where you were and where you are now.

Keep your road as your map to guide you, to help you see how far you have come. Keep adding to it as you walk your road, write down every step that gives you hope and encouragement. Let it sustain you on the bad days and inspire you to keep moving as you heal beyond birth trauma.

BEYOND

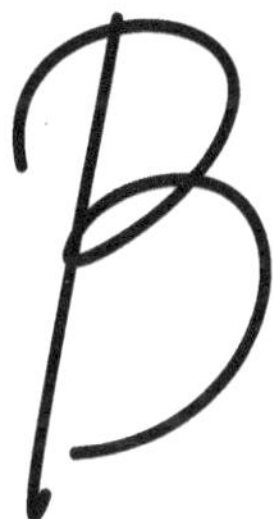

4

B - BIRTH MATTERS

"Your story is your gift of healing."

"Everyone told me that my birth didn't matter because I had my baby, but it did matter, it mattered to me."
Jo

I look around the room, there are mums and babies everywhere. I look at their faces, smiling and happy. They are chatting, discussing if their little one is sleeping through the night or sitting up yet. I stare at them, looking for a trace or a flicker that may show deep down they are suffering too. You see I'm suffering, fear exists in me that won't let go, I watch my daughter sitting nearby playing with a small toy in her hand, I'm trying hard not to react, to run over and check she is ok every few minutes. I know she is, and I know we are both okay now, but still the 'what if' is there playing like a movie in my mind.

Yes, we are lucky to be here, I'm lucky the doctors were able to save me as my life blood poured from me, and lucky that my daughter was born in a hospital that had a neonatal unit with medical equipment to save her too. But I don't feel lucky, because a part of me changed forever that night, and more of me was stolen in the weeks that followed. Those I trusted to care for me treated me with unkindness and cruelty, like I didn't matter, and wasn't worth their concern, not even their pity.

So here I was, a shell of my former self, in a bubble of fear, anxiety and worry. Yet my lips felt glued together because I could not voice the pain I was feeling or the thoughts that were holding my mind captive. I couldn't put into words the visions I saw in the dark of night or the constant worries that crept into everything I did, and everywhere I went, till it became painful to do even the simplest things. No one saw behind the mask I wore and how I winced every time someone went near my daughter, or she went anywhere without me. But keeping the mask in place was becoming harder, and when it became all too much, and I could no longer stop it from slipping, I would sink into the darkness, fear gripping me, and I felt so alone. Birth trauma had changed my life, it had changed my future, it had changed me.

Why Birth Matters

The Birth of your baby matters, it matters because it significantly impacts you and your life. Birth is the start of your relationship with a new human being that you have made, grown and nurtured for over nine months. It is a time of hopes and dreams, a new journey that is scary as well as exciting, the future ahead unwritten and unsure.

There have been many months of waiting, an expectation of how the birth of your baby would be, that was thought about, anticipated and planned. Those months spent planning come down to this, welcoming into the world your beautiful new baby. But what happens when the birth of your baby is difficult? What happens when birth leaves you feeling let down and distressed? What if instead of being the happy event you had longed for it has left you feeling traumatised?

When you lose a much-wanted birth experience it can leave a void inside you that you struggle to understand. It can also in its wake leave you full of unwanted emotions, including sadness, anger, guilt and disappointment. All that you have planned and prepared for your baby's birth over many months even years, now lays in tatters. The loss of this is very real like a thief has come and stolen something precious from you. Your baby may be here, but how they arrived may have affected you beyond comprehension. This matters and can be deeply distressing to new parents.

There can be an attitude in society that it doesn't matter how your baby was born, but it does matter, to you. Family and friends while well-meaning, can be quick to dismiss any feelings you may have that suggest your birth didn't go as you wanted it to. Often it is said to new parents that a healthy baby is all that matters. However, the loss of how you wanted your birth to be, can be a source of great trauma.

It may be that the circumstances surrounding the birth meant the loss of a peaceful birth experience, instead leaving you feeling anxious or disappointed. Sometimes birth becomes an emergency situation where your life or that of your baby is threatened. It could be that you struggle with any medical interventions that happened during your birth. Maybe you needed help to cope with the pain, or a long labour left you feeling exhausted and needing help to deliver your baby. It can be hard to come to terms with the changes or any interventions that happened especially as most women will desire to labour and birth without them. The loss of a wanted birth experience whatever that may be really does matter.

At times babies are born early or sick and need the support of a neonatal unit. Again this can lead to many difficult emotions. When a pregnancy ends suddenly, often due to a mother or baby being at risk, this can be very distressing. The loss of those last weeks, not being able to attend antenatal classes, or prepare at home for your baby can leave a feeling of loss and disappointment. Many women will voice that they feel they have somehow failed to keep their baby safe or that their bodies have failed because their baby was born early. Guilt can often be an emotion that creeps in, as can anger and frustration.

The neonatal unit itself can be a difficult environment, with alarms, medical equipment and tiny bundles covered in tubes and wires. Constant worry about your baby as well as trying to recover yourself from birth, while also juggling home and even other children can be a huge amount of stress. The daily threat and worry over your baby's survival, as well as the many medical procedures needed to keep babies safe is hard to manage, especially when born very early. Many families can spend weeks or months in a neonatal unit before bringing their baby home. It's not uncommon therefore for parents to show signs of distress and even symptoms of post-traumatic distress disorder (PTSD) after having a baby in neonatal.

Sadly some experience poor care during birth. You may feel let down by those over your care. Your trust may have been broken and left you reeling in the face of unkind actions, cruel words or any neglect that you have experienced, be it physically or emotionally. You may have felt a loss of control, dignity or privacy, leaving you feeling vulnerable and confused. There may have been a lack of information given to you that has left you unsure about certain aspects of your birth or care. Or you may feel you were not listened to or your choices were not respected or were even disregarded or overlooked. You may feel that medical procedures were done without your consent or proper explanation or that you were left with no choice. You may feel that the choices offered did not reflect the true situation or that coercion was used.

You may feel that you suffered discrimination in your birth due to your skin colour, religion, social or economic situation, gender or culture. This means your experience has been tainted and left you feeling vulnerable.

Poor care can take many forms from actual physical harm to emotional and psychological harm. In my experience of caring for families after a difficult birth, poor care is often the hardest aspect. You place your trust in healthcare professionals to keep you safe not only physically but emotionally. Sometimes the care given is so lacking it leads to medical mistakes that cause great harm to a woman or her baby, even the need for further medical treatment. In some cases, it has meant the loss of a woman and/or her baby. For families in the aftermath of poor care, the impact can be devastating and life-changing. Often families will voice that they then also struggled to access support or the answers as to what happened, including the taking of responsibility in cases of medical neglect.

Good care is a fundamentally important part of the maternity journey, especially birth and can be the difference between leaving families emotionally well or emotionally traumatised. Even in the most challenging of situations, even when sadly babies are lost during birth when the care given is compassionate and kind it can serve as a buffer to trauma.

Of course, none of this may be your experience. It could be that on paper your birth to others appears to have been a positive experience with nothing obviously traumatic. However, for you, it may have felt deeply traumatic leaving you feeling numb, confused, even isolated, unable to voice how you truly feel.

I once supported a woman who had struggled with her birth experience for many months. She broke down before me exclaiming that she had seemingly had the 'perfect birth' so why did she feel traumatised? She voiced how her partner and family had told everyone how amazing it was and she felt silenced not wishing to burst their bubble. She blamed herself, feeling ashamed that she felt so affected by her baby's birth, especially when others were telling her how lucky she was. This led to her suffering greatly with her mental health and struggling to bond with her baby. The reality was there were lots of reasons why she felt her birth was traumatic that were individual to her, they were all valid and needed the acknowledgement they deserved.

Yes, birth trauma is complex, just as we are complex as individuals. Never should we presume to know what birth feels like for someone else, instead we must always listen to understand their reality. It isn't what others think or feel about your birth, it is how you feel that matters. For me it was a combination of things, my daughter was born early, the journey of neonatal, medical complications, poor care and lack of support in the postnatal period all added to my feeling traumatised.

In the many years I've listened to families the complexity of birth trauma is what stands out. Sadly the view of many can be that the birth experience doesn't matter, as long as the woman and her baby are medically safe. This view can cause those who experience a difficult birth to feel that to speak up, is making a fuss or not being grateful for having a healthy baby. The result can be the silencing of painful emotions and memories, and these are sometimes then carried for years, locked away, but still causing pain. I have had grandmothers contact me for support after carrying for years the pain of their births, often after seeing their daughters or granddaughters have children of their own. We cannot underestimate how much the birth experience matters.

If you feel traumatised from your birth experience you may feel isolated, as those around you may not understand why. It can make you feel guilty or somehow weaker than other women for being unable to cope with your feelings about your birth experience. I find this the hardest of all because the women I meet who struggle each day with birth trauma have no idea how strong they really are. You may feel pressured to just 'get over' the birth and as we have already said often well-meaning friends and family may say things such as 'at least you are ok now, and you have a healthy baby, so that's what matters'. This only seeks to confound your feelings and make you feel more isolated. This is silencing because the more you attempt to say how you feel when this is met with dismissal, however well intended, it causes you to try to bury those feelings and thus prevents healing.

Birth matters too because birth trauma can damage relationships with your partner, family members and friends. You may feel no one understands, that they can't see your struggle with what has happened to you. Many women have said to me they feel anger towards their partner and/or family for feeling left or abandoned, for not being heard or ignored, or for in some ways allowing the events of their birth to happen.

Birth trauma damages relationships because we are naturally attuned to seek connection but trauma sends us into a self-protective mode which means trust and connection become difficult. Marriages can break, friendships can be lost as birth trauma wreaks havoc in the lives of those it touches. When trust is lost rebuilding this can be difficult, when trauma is the cause it can feel impossible. When struggling after a difficult birth you can feel like walls have been built around you that no one can break through.

As we saw in the chapter *What is Birth Trauma*, it can also affect the sexual aspects of your relationship. It may be the fear of further pregnancies which can become so great that you are both physically and emotionally unable to engage in any sexual contact. Especially if you have experienced physical damage from medical procedures such as an episiotomy, sexual activity can again feel impossible. Any intimacy can indeed feel impossible, even to be held or touched by a loved one as you struggle to feel safe or trusting of anyone. This again can cause many difficult emotions and impact precious relationships.

Depending on the nature of the trauma you may feel unable to have needed medical appointments. Often so broken is the trust especially after poor care that seeking any support from healthcare professionals is impossible. I know in the aftermath of my birth trauma I was struggling to trust anyone who was a healthcare professional. I hated attending baby clinics and if I was visited at home would have sleepless nights for days. I felt the need to protect my daughter and would question everything that was advised me about her care. When it came to myself, health anxiety was something I battled with but seeking medical help felt out of the question so broken was my trust in the medical profession.

You may feel that birth trauma has caused you to struggle to bond with your baby, maybe you feel triggered by your baby, bringing back painful memories, leaving you struggling to care for and love your baby due to the trauma you feel. Or you may feel disassociated from everything and everyone around you in order to cope with your experience and the aftermath, including your baby. It's not uncommon to wish others to care for your baby, or to believe that your baby is better with someone else. This can leave you berating yourself for not feeling the rush of love you expected, and it can be easy to become consumed with the belief you aren't a good parent.

Birth trauma can also impact things such as breastfeeding, again causing you to feel that you have somehow failed if this was something you wanted to do. Of course, when serious physical recovery is also needed just caring for a newborn can feel completely overwhelming and for some has been impossible.

You may also feel overly anxious about your baby's health and well-being and constantly worry about every aspect of caring for your newborn. You may be anxious that something will happen to your baby, and as such avoid anything that you deem to be a risk. Experiencing intrusive thoughts of harm coming to your baby or even that you may be the cause of the harm can be common after birth trauma and can be a source of great distress.

Women who have lost a baby during birth may experience not only devastation but overwhelming guilt, they may feel like it was their fault, that they somehow failed their baby or that they should somehow have prevented it. Sadly, lack of support after loss during birth is common with many voicing after the loss of a baby that they were left to get on with it. This means trauma has space to take root and grow. After the excitement of pregnancy and the hopes of having a new baby, dreams are dashed to pieces and families are left with pain, heartbreak and sorrow. Many families struggle to come to terms with their loss, many feeling despair, guilt, confusion and anguish. Empty arms are a constant reminder of their loss and of stolen memories

The reality of birth trauma for many is feeling like you have no voice, are misunderstood or weak, many will seek to hide their true suffering and 'carry on', the weight of trauma bearing down on them crushing hope, light and happiness as they try desperately to cling to normality. Everyday life can soon become hard and just coping day to day can feel impossible and overwhelming. Physical health too may suffer as the effects of trauma ravage you mentally. Lack of sleep, trouble eating and constant anxiety all take their toll. Flashbacks may take you back to the event reliving moments, even smells and conversations, causing great distress and anxiety.

Yes, a traumatic birth can change everything. Birth matters on so many levels, it is an experience you will remember your whole life. Birth matters, it mattered to me and it matters to you.

You Matter

The truth is your birth experience matters and how you feel about your birth experience also matters. The acknowledgement of this is very important and the first step in healing. So, while others may try to tell you to forget what has happened, to move on and find joy in being a parent, this can often lead to hurt remaining and healing left undone.

It matters because when we are traumatised, we often superimpose how we feel onto everything around us, it then becomes hard to know what is reality and what is trauma. We see the world differently, through a trauma lens so to speak and so understanding that our birth matters, that the trauma we feel is valid is vital.

I remember the first few days at home with my daughter. We had been in the hospital for nearly five weeks, and home felt unfamiliar. I felt like I had been hit by something so massive that I had no idea how to even start processing it. Everything felt like a daze, almost like I was not part of reality. I wondered if everyone felt like I did after birth, lost and scared. I would watch those around me laughing and cooing over my daughter, irritated that they were so carefree, so seemingly unaffected. Sometimes I would think about how the scenes would then have played out had I not survived. It tormented me, and I felt so alone. The trauma lens had me very focused on, in fact, zoomed in on what was now a world of anguish and fear.

As the days turned into weeks and then months what I found the hardest was the silence I felt forced into. It was as if the weeks I had spent in the hospital hadn't happened, the great unspoken event that was now ignored. No one spoke about it, not the nurse who came each day to give me my iron injections, not those I loved who chatted about the mundane things of daily life. I wanted to speak, I wanted to cry and scream and shout. I wanted to let out the pain and the hurt that made my chest feel like it was going to explode. Yet even the times when I did try to say how I was feeling I was met with denial. Well-meant words telling me to let it go, to no longer think about it, that I had to think about the future and my baby, this only silenced me more.

As time crept by my silencing led to deeper pain. I started to feel that it was me that was at fault. After all, women gave birth every day and were fine, weren't they? How weak was I that I couldn't pull myself together? Why couldn't I make the visions that visited me at night stop? How could I be so ungrateful that I was not able to be happy to have my beautiful daughter? Yes, I must be the defective one, the one that was to blame. So, the pain spread through me, deeper, causing more guilt, more pain, and more anguish. I felt like my birth didn't matter to anyone, that I had nearly died and so had my daughter, but it was simply ignored. I felt like I had been through the most difficult time of my life but it was of no regard to anyone else. It made me feel worthless, that my feelings and pain were worthless. That I simply didn't matter.

The truth was I did matter and so do you. Trauma isn't just an event that happened and has now gone, it leaves an imprint on your mind and body. It changes how you think, how you feel, and how you function. Often this means you will live as if the trauma is still going on, on edge and fearful of what may happen next.

Trauma means it can be difficult to determine if any situation is dangerous or safe, in a constant state of scanning, ready to spring into action if needed. Even normal situations can cause anxiety. Years ago I had a woman voice to me that she found changing her own baby's nappy to be immensely anxiety-inducing, but she had no idea why, after talking through her birth it became clear that it was during her baby's nappy change that she collapsed due to sudden severe blood loss. While she hadn't made this connection her brain had and as a result now caused her to feel anxiety each time she needed to do this basic care for her baby.

Triggers can be everywhere and trying to live each day with the impact of trauma is exhausting. Trauma doesn't just go away, instead, you need the right help and support to help it heal. I like to think of it as if our safe world has been shattered, like a beautiful picture now lying in pieces. Our world no longer feels safe and the picture we had broken. So how do we begin to heal?

Part of healing is helping the mind and body relearn that the danger has now passed and that instead of looking through the lens of trauma, you need to come back to the reality of now. That the world can be safe again and you can rebuild your picture. However, you cannot begin to heal and find relief until your trauma is acknowledged and validated and you see the truth of what you are struggling with. This begins with the truth that your birth experience matters and so do you.

Being able to acknowledge your experience and the impact on you, is the first step towards healing. Like an open wound cannot just be ignored, so too when your birth experience wounds you it matters that the wound is acknowledged, and support is given to help it heal.

When birth causes trauma it affects everything. It cannot be ignored, if you try to it will continue to keep reminding you that it is there. Birth matters and so do you. When you feel that your birth has been difficult it must be acknowledged both by you and those around you.

Being heard

Whenever I speak to women who come to me for support, they voice that they often feel unheard, holding in difficult emotions that are causing them so much pain. Sometimes this pain has been carried for many years. You need to be heard to heal!

On the first day of my training as a Birth Buddy, there were about 15 of us some colleagues whom I had worked with for a while, excited to learn more about helping families on their maternity journey. The session in the afternoon was about our own birth experiences and how processing them was important for us to be able to care for the women whom we would be advocating for. As we went around the room, I listened to the others telling various versions of their birth stories. When it got to me I felt the words stick in my throat, I never lifted my eyes from the floor as in a quiet voice I recounted my edited version of my daughter's birth. I'm sure that it all tumbled out, jumbled up and not very coherent and when I stopped speaking I looked up to very shocked faces. My tutor whom I admired and looked up to, had eyes filled with tears and everyone around me was shaking their heads in disbelief. In a sudden wave, a sea of arms engulfed me, and tears fell from eyes that had too long been dry. This was the first time that I had been allowed to openly speak about what had happened, and the first time I had been listened to, without interruption, judgment and dismissal. That day proved to be a huge step in my healing. A profound day that meant so much.

My tutor kept me behind, and we talked at length over the next few weeks about how I felt about all that I had been through. No answers were given to me, only the space to talk, in safety and empathy. It was so powerful to finally be heard, to let out all my pain and to feel cared for. It also gave me the chance to acknowledge that my birth mattered. That what I had lost mattered. That how I felt mattered. That I mattered. Yes, I had a healthy baby eventually, but it mattered that our journey to get there had been hard. I had been emotionally battered and bruised, and while my physical healing had taken many months, mentally my healing was nowhere near done. What I needed was the space to heal mentally too. You cannot underestimate how important this is, to have space to acknowledge what happened to you and for someone to hold that safe space for you.

When I admitted that my birth experience mattered it opened the way to understanding why. I started to work out what it was that mattered to me, what I had lost, what I was struggling with and why. An example of this was having the space to then be able to grieve the loss of those precious 'firsts,' the first cuddle, first nappy change and first feed. These mattered to me and they were lost because of the circumstances of our birth. Nothing could give those things back to me, it hurt and that was ok. I had a right to feel cheated and robbed of such precious things. Knowing these mattered along with so many other things, allowed me to start to heal and with that some peace started to return.

Another part of acknowledging your birth matters is regaining a sense of stability and safety. This can take time. After birth trauma you can feel overwhelmed, anxious and terrified. Trauma rocks you to your very core. It questions everything including your own mortality. The world can now feel like a scary place and like you are living in constant fear. Every day can be a battle while your mind is on high alert for any impending danger. This can mean that things you once didn't even notice, are now perceived as threats. The emotional reactions that you may experience can leave you feeling out of control. Anything can trigger you sending you back to strong feelings you struggle to manage. These are emotional flashbacks and they need to be acknowledged and understood. To gain back a feeling of safety means knowing that you have been through trauma and as such your sense of the world has changed. It also means knowing that the emotions that come back when triggered are not about now, but about what happened in the past. It was the past that felt unsafe, and now you will need to believe you are safe again.

It's good to acknowledge too that if you have also had a difficult pregnancy this means that living with constant anxiety has been your reality now for many months. When I looked back, I realised that it wasn't just the birth that had affected me but the loss of my daughter's twin at 8 weeks and then a difficult pregnancy where I was terrified that I would lose my now only baby. In truth, my world hadn't been safe for a very long time and this state of fear and anxiety had become my 'norm'.

Feeling safe again can take a long time to achieve. The body and the mind need time to come down, so to speak, from this new place of fear and to learn that safety is possible again. This I will talk about later on in the book.

Knowing that your birth matters, how it has affected you and that your feelings are valid can support you to feel stable and in control. How? Once you understand that what you have been through is important, you can then make the choice to find the help you deserve and need. It allows the taking back of some of the control that often trauma can strip away, in the knowledge that you can find healing and safety once again.

It also means that you can have an awareness of how the trauma is impacting you daily and how when it isn't acknowledged and given the space it needs to heal, can then start to define you, leaving you without peace and struggling to cope. Just as we mentioned earlier like a physical wound needs the right care to heal, so do emotional wounds. You cannot just ignore them otherwise they will infect you, festering away and before long start oozing poison that will invade every aspect of your life.

It's all about you

It doesn't matter what anyone thinks, or tells you, what matters is how you feel. This step is when you start to take back what was stolen from you, where you make the choice that your trauma is not going to define you. It means knowing that you deserve to be heard and that all you have gone through needs to be acknowledged. You no longer have to feel silenced, ashamed, guilty or to blame. It means owning your experience, with all the pain, knowing this will be the start of your journey to healing. You will need to be brave, leaving doubt behind while seeking to look forward with new hope. This will not be easy but it is possible. This means owing your birth story.

Some may not support your new voice especially as you try to wade through what happened and may try to tell you that you need to try and move on. This can be painful as you seek to heal.

It may mean that you will seek to find answers about what happened in your birth, which could mean talking to those over your care to understand what really happened. It may also mean admitting that you need to ask for help and support as you navigate the days, weeks, or months ahead. This may be practical ways as well as through therapy from the right services.

Owning your story, and saying that it matters are the first steps on your road to healing. They are small steps, but powerful ones. Do not underestimate them. If you are sitting now holding this book in your hands, say it out loud. MY BIRTH MATTERS, I MATTER.

Yes, birth matters, especially YOUR experience of birth. The road to healing starts with the small step of understanding why your birth matters, how your birth experience has impacted you, how it has made you feel, and that it is important. Denying or fighting how you feel doesn't help you to heal, it holds you back from taking those first steps as you try to walk your road.

Remember from the previous chapter we saw how healing comes from within? This starts with the awareness of what it is that you need to heal and this is found in knowing that your birth experience matters.

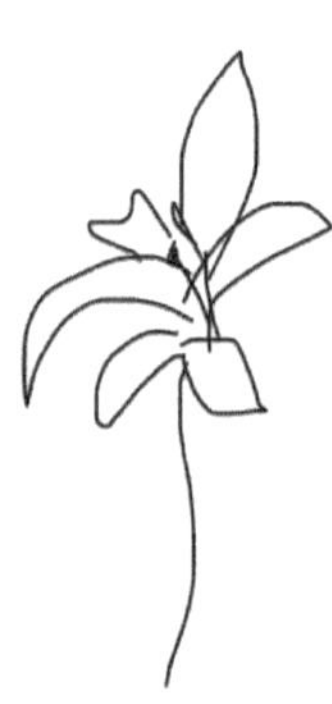

A reflection for you.

Once I felt heard something changed, my experience started to relinquish its control. One thing that helped me immensely was journaling. I started to write down what had happened. Sometimes it was memories, snapshots of moments in time, and sometimes words of others or how I felt. I would write it as it came to me, in the pages of my notebook. It was hard and sometimes the words written would be smeared by the tears that fell as I wrote. Slowly over time I wrote pages of what I had lost, what it had cost me, how it was impacting me and even moments of light in all the darkness.

One day I sat and read it all back, a timeline of all that had been my experience. I then saw it with new eyes. I saw the raw pain, the anguish and how I had been treated and my perspective changed. I wasn't weak, I wasn't at fault, I had been through a traumatic experience and that's why I was suffering. Most of all I saw that my birth experience mattered!

When you put into words the thoughts in your head it enables you to understand better what happened or how you are feeling. It also allows you during times when thoughts may be overwhelming to let them out, writing them down and then leaving them there when you close the book. So, when you are ready and when the time is right, try it.

Try it.

- Find a notebook that has meaning to you. It may have a beautiful picture or a meaningful quote on its cover.
- Write about your deepest thoughts, feelings or memories about why your birth experience matters. Let them flow. Do not force them but let them come naturally. There are no time constraints. It may be each day, or weeks

apart, it's up to you. You can write down your feelings or what happened, as a story, as a letter to someone, or even as pictures or doodles.

- You may find that facing how you feel can be distressing especially at first, so take some time for yourself to manage any distress you may feel using ways that are supportive of you. (I would remind myself it was hard but part of my journey to healing)
- Do not worry about grammar or spelling, they are not important. What is important is being able to express yourself from the heart.
- You may with time wish to share some of your writing with loved ones to help them understand how you are feeling and this can open up the way for honest, heartfelt conversations that also support healing.
- Take time to ponder what you have written, to truly over time come to understand what about your birth mattered. Let these guide you to see what things need support to heal.

For me when I finally saw that my birth mattered, I saw that I mattered. That I deserved to be heard, to be helped and supported to find healing.

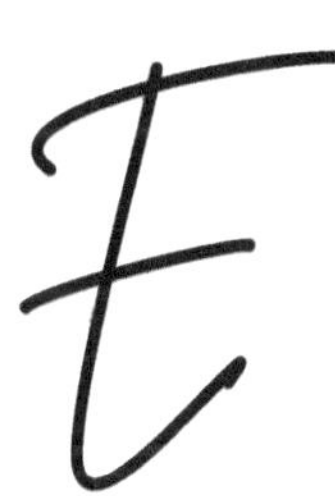

5

E - EXPLORE YOUR EXPERIENCE

"Out of suffering have emerged the strongest souls, the most massive characters are seared with scars."
Khalil Gibran

"Everyone said how wonderful my birth was, but that wasn't how I had experienced it. I felt like I couldn't say how it had affected me, and I was scared of what everyone would think of me if I told them how I truly felt."
Amy

Your birth experience is your experience and yours alone. How you feel about your birth experience is individual to you. Only you know your birth and how you experienced it.

Regardless of who else was with you, it is how you experienced it that matters. It may be that your birth was outwardly a very traumatic experience, or it may be that to others, your birth experience appeared to be good or even positive. Regardless of how others may feel about the birth of your baby, what matters is how you feel.

All the experiences that you go through in life affect and impact you. The birth of your baby is no different. When birth is traumatic it can change you beyond all recognition and can ultimately also change your view of the world around you. The world can suddenly be a place where you see danger everywhere and you can feel as if you are constantly on high alert. When this happens, it can also change how you react to situations you can find yourself in. Things that once were easy or you loved to do, can now be hard and no longer enjoyable. Strong emotions may overtake you and you may feel that they are out of your control. When trauma happens, you can question every aspect of life and you may struggle in the aftermath with how to come to terms with what has happened.

Of course, when it comes to birth trauma not only is it the birth that impacts you, but also the transition to being a new parent with a new baby. This tiny person who needs you and who you are responsible for 24 hours a day, seven days a week while being amazing, can also leave you feeling overwhelmed. Sometimes when new parents find transitioning to being parents hard, it is assumed that it is just the normal process of having a baby, and most times this is true, yet it isn't always explored whether their birth experience has played a part in why they may be struggling.

Often after a difficult birth, you can try to push it to the back of your mind, trying to forget it and carry on as if nothing has happened. The focus of course is also on trying to recover and care for your new baby. Life is busy with nappies, feeding, sleepless nights, the endless stream of visitors and just trying to get through each day and night.

When trauma occurs it doesn't just go away, however much we wish it and often will manifest itself in many ways, especially in relation to our emotions. When this happens due to birth you may find that you are filled with anxious thoughts or experiencing low mood, even if you have never had this before. Or you may feel anger or other unwelcome emotions that you don't understand or know why they are here. Sometimes it can be your relationship with your baby or partner that is affected as we have already seen. Or it can be that life in general just feels like it's all too much, and you may suddenly feel you are spinning out of control.

Difficult emotions, difficulties in your relationships, struggling with your mental health or bonding with your baby however don't always get linked to a traumatic birth either by yourself or those around you. Exploring your journey of pregnancy and birth and how it has made you feel can often show if there are any links between what happened and the emotions and sensations you may be experiencing now. Many times I have seen parents being labelled as anxious or depressed yet their birth experience is ignored. In reality, a difficult maternity journey is often the reason.

Of course, it's not just emotions that parents may experience after a difficult birth but overwhelming physical reactions too. Why?

Birth trauma is much more than the story of what happened to you. The emotions and physical sensations that you experienced during your birth became imprinted on you. These are often experienced after the event not so much as memories, but as an emotional and very real physical reaction. This is because the emotional part of your brain expresses itself in very physical ways, such as a pounding heart, be it with excitement or fear. Of course when the sensation is unpleasant your natural reaction is to avoid anything that makes you feel that way, including your birth experience. So, it can be hard to explore and own your experience or even to admit or accept it. This can be especially hard if everyone around you is saying it wasn't that bad or they feel it was different to how you experienced it.

It may be hard also because exploring your experience can bring up unwanted feelings, feelings that you may have tried hard not to feel, such as guilt, disappointment or grief. Our natural response to anything that brings up unwanted emotions is to push it away, avoiding it at all costs. Even if the rational part of our brain can understand why these responses are there, it doesn't change how it makes us feel physically.

It can be hard also if the way you planned to give birth wasn't possible and you feel the loss of a much-wanted experience. There can be many conflicting emotions after the loss of the birth you wanted, feeling happy that your baby is here, but feeling sad about how it happened. It can be hard though to express to anyone that you may be finding it difficult when birth is something that is viewed as a wonderful event to be celebrated. This again can lead to avoidance of exploring your experience, leading to you struggling silently with how it has affected you.

Another reason why you can struggle to explore your birth experience is that we are surrounded by visions of how birth is depicted. From the extremes of television shows to blissful images on social media, birth can be portrayed on a wide spectrum from sheer joy to terror. It can be difficult to find where your experience fits on this spectrum and with so many expectations around how birth should be, accepting, exploring and owning your own experience can be a challenge. Yet what is the reality of birth?

Don't Compare

Birth is complex, raw, primal, life-changing, unpredictable and individual, to you. Your birth experience is just that, yours. There can be the temptation however to compare your experience. You may compare it to the expectations and experiences of others or you may compare it to the expectations of how you believe it should have been. In fact, when it comes to all aspects of pregnancy, birth and parenting you may find yourself comparing what you are experiencing to every other parent you know or come in contact with. When you are comparing your experiences with those of others you can greatly add to your anxiety and feelings of sadness around your birth experience.

When it comes to birth there is much complexity. As we said before it is as individual as you are and yet this is often not accounted for. Comparing birth experiences can take many different approaches. Many women have said to me that they have felt their birth was not as bad as others they have heard of and so feel ashamed that they feel traumatised. Others have voiced that they struggle to come to terms with what has happened because they believe they have failed in some way or even failed their babies. Others have felt distress for not having what is termed a 'normal birth', or that they haven't birthed the right way. Others have voiced that they feel as if they haven't given birth at all and feel robbed of the experience. Remember we also in the last chapter discussed how you can see things through a trauma lens so comparing your experience and yourself to others can become a favourite past-time.

It doesn't just apply to the birth experience itself, but this can also be the case as you begin your journey as a new parent. After my daughter's birth, my expectation of myself was to be the perfect mother. I struggled with the fact that for days we had been separated after her birth and the pain tore at me causing massive guilt. It felt like I needed to in some way make up for this and now do everything perfectly. I put huge pressure on myself as to how I thought I should be as a parent for her. My trauma lens was making me doubt my abilities as a mother, it also made me set unrealistic expectations for myself that I could never meet. The more I couldn't in my eyes 'match up', the more of a failure I felt, until all I saw was the things I thought I wasn't doing, instead of all the things I was doing.

My traumatic birth left me comparing my birth and myself with others and trying to live up to what I believed I should be as a mother, instead of seeing the reality. The reality was that I had been through a birth that had nearly taken my life and that of my baby that had been damaged both physically and emotionally.

My reality had been five weeks in the hospital and neonatal unit and huge medical complications to heal. What I needed was time and rest to recover. However, my expectations were to be back to the old me, doing everything as before, that my birth should have somehow not affected me. The more I compared, the more I needed to put on a mask and pretend to everyone that I was okay. I became compulsive at cleaning, had huge anxiety about my daughter's health and well-being, and was driven by the need to be the perfect mother. I was trying to compensate for the birth and it became a coping strategy to try and dull down how I was feeling. Sadly no one linked this to my birth experience, including myself. Instead, I was made to feel like I was a 'neurotic mother' as one doctor called me, who was overprotective and not adjusting to motherhood well. I began to believe that the fault lay with me, that I just couldn't cope like other women did. This in turn drove me to look at other families even more, longing to be just like them and the distorted view I had of what family life should be. This led to a dark downward spiral of self-doubt, guilt and anguish.

In truth, it wasn't that I couldn't cope, or that I wasn't a good mother but that I had been through a traumatic event and I was trying to cope with it the best way I could, what I needed was support to heal and recover.

How else may you compare your birth? Over the years I've had women contact me who during their pregnancy had attended antenatal classes where the preparation was to support having as natural a birth as possible. This they have then struggled with when their birth led to the need for interventions or took a different path. Many voiced that they felt unable to return to the group they had been attending before or sadly even felt unwelcome to return because they hadn't experienced what was an expected natural birth. This led to them feeling that they had in some way failed, or not met the expectations of others or themselves. In turn, feeling this way has meant them not wanting to own their experience. They compare what they hoped for, with what happened, and put the blame on themselves, feeling that they must have done something wrong for their birth to have been so difficult. They may then feel that someone else's experience is better or could have been achievable had they just done something differently.

Others have voiced the pain they feel at hearing friends or relatives talk about a birth that has been positive or pain-free when their experience of birth has been anything but this. Comparing their experience causes so much hurt it has led them to distance themselves from others due to the painful feelings this invokes, often damaging friendships but feeling helpless to prevent this.

Many have been led to believe that birth is only positive if done a certain way, so feel guilty when this isn't possible. Others have voiced that they have struggled to accept the way their birth progressed because they have felt ashamed to say that they needed pain relief or interventions or have chosen to birth a certain way, for fear of what others may think of them.

It always makes me so sad to see women compare their birth experiences and feel somehow lesser as a result. Remember, no one knows your reality other than you, the person who has experienced the birth. Only you know how you feel and how it has impacted you. If you are struggling know that you are not alone. How do you know that the woman sitting across from you or that you met in the park or is smiling in a picture on Facebook isn't struggling too? I can't even begin to recount how many women have told me about some aspect of their birth that they have found difficult.

The reality is that pregnancy and birth are a complex journey that many find hard. I've spoken to women who have endured the most traumatic of births and yet have voiced that they feel they are somehow weak and a failure. How can we view anyone who has gone through such difficult circumstances as weak or a failure? It always makes my heart hurt to see women racked with pain believing they have somehow failed in birthing their babies when in reality it is very much the opposite. Birth takes courage and strength, and women show how amazing they are in often very difficult and challenging circumstances.

Comparing your experience isn't helpful in healing from a difficult birth experience. It can instead intensify feelings that cause distress. As we said above birth is individual to you, in fact, every birth is individual to that woman and that baby. Both my experiences of birth were as unique as my daughters are. What can be helpful instead is to reflect on your own experience of birth and what it means to you. It has been your journey and only you know how it has informed how you feel.

So remember your experience is individual to you and healing means that instead of comparing your birth, you gently own your experience, even though it may have not been the experience you had hoped for. Exploring it, how it has made you feel and why it matters to you will help you find ways to process and understand it which can help you find healing.

What is your reality?

Another reason for exploring your experience is to find your truth and the reality of what happened. What does this mean? You may think that you can get rid of your trauma or control it by silencing it. You may try to hide from what was the reality especially if it causes you to feel unwanted emotions such as anger or shame. However, by silencing your trauma it will be hard to journey your road to healing, it also reinforces the awful isolation that often accompanies it. If you seek to keep the secrets of your trauma, you will wage an inner war that will eat away at you, your identity, beliefs and worth.

When you are instead able to voice and acknowledge your experience, when you feel listened to and have an awareness of how trauma is affecting you, this supports healing. It allows you to gain perspective on what happened and it also allows you to find freedom. That is freedom from trying to avoid anything that may trigger emotions that arise due to not seeing the truth of what your experience meant to you. This includes accepting the reality of your experience.

I know that for a long time, I denied and downplayed my birth experience. Part of this was not having the space to be honest about how I had been affected, but part of it was also that most of my trauma was due to poor care, even cruel treatment by the healthcare staff whom I trusted to care for me. I guess in my mind it was hard to believe that individuals could cause such suffering, show such cruelty or ultimately not care about me or what had happened to me. I also had a hard time accepting that I allowed people to treat me so badly, that I believe I hadn't advocated for myself or my baby, that I allowed myself to be vulnerable and worse still that this then impacted my relationship with my baby. It became easier to stay silent and also blame myself. This in turn prevented me from walking my road to healing.

The road to healing includes seeing the reality of your experience and this can be brutal and painful. It may mean that you also accept the truth that your birth wasn't a happy, joyous welcoming of your baby into the world, but instead, a deeply distressing and traumatic event which has left you now wondering how you will ever enjoy life again. It can mean the accepting of things that meant so much to you that were lost. It can mean embracing much disappointment and sadness.

Another aspect of this can be the narrative you have of your birth which is the 'public story' you tell others and the reality of what actually happened. This can be especially hard as you may create a story that you feel is what others want to hear or out of fear of telling your 'truth'. However for healing to take place your public story needs to meet with the reality of what was your experience and this allows for reconciling how you have been affected. This doesn't mean recounting every detail to those you meet, but it can be as simple as honestly sharing that it was a difficult time and as such you are taking the needed time to recover.

What about your reality when it comes to expectations? Are you expecting too much of yourself both regarding the birth and also being a parent? Do you need to be kinder to yourself and know your limitations?

My reality was I expected too much of myself and also had a trauma lens view of what others expected of me. I had advice thrown at me from everywhere, parents, grandparents, friends, healthcare professionals and so on. In striving to make up for believing that my body failed and the trauma that was my daughter's birth I tried to please everyone around me. I strove to be perfect which also meant that I believed I needed to gain the acceptance of others so that they believed me to be perfect too. I also expected the most ridiculous things of myself both physically and emotionally. I can remember only two days after being discharged from the hospital there was a function for family and friends and of course, I believed I was obligated to attend. I was battered and bruised, my blood iron levels so low I still had trouble standing and breathing. Yet I painted my face, adorned my clothes and made myself attend while being dizzy and unsteady on my feet, plus a tiny 4lb baby in tow! I was bombarded with questions about the birth and everyone was clamouring trying to look at and touch my daughter. I felt like a rabbit in the headlights, but also in a cage, unable to leave, trapped. It set me back massively and the first time that I truly felt the knife-like stab of panic that made me want to run and hide, to lock me and my daughter away and never see anyone again.

Hindsight is a wonderful thing and I see now that I allowed the expectations of others, to set my expectations for me, which was detrimental to my well-being. I was physically and emotionally unwell, I needed time to rest, heal and recover. I wasn't prepared for the questions around my birth, I also didn't realise how trauma had made me so hyper-vigilance about my daughter. The panic I felt was my brain trying to protect me, where it perceived danger, it was my soul screaming at me that this was too much and overwhelming.

This is where I was able to gain the perspective I mentioned above. The reality was, and it took me a long time to realise this, was that what I had needed in those early days and weeks after my daughter's birth was to just be kind to myself. To allow myself the time to heal physically, to process all that we had been through and to understand that mentally I was struggling. I had suffered massive trauma and as such needed help and support to enable me to start the road to healing, everything else could wait.

Another reality that came with hindsight was that all my baby needed was my love and to be cared for as best I could. Perfection was unattainable, striving to reach perfection only set me up to fail and left me feeling I was letting everyone down. It was an impossible expectation that I had set myself. I didn't need to make up for my traumatic birth, I only needed to heal from it. As for my daughter what she needed was a healthy mum physically and emotionally not a social butterfly or a perfectly clean house.

Another part of finding your reality and indeed comparing your birth is when you feel that your experience hasn't been that bad and as such downplay or dismiss how you feel. You cannot compare experiences. What one woman may find traumatic, another may not. There are so many reasons that birth is perceived to be traumatic, too many and too complex that this alone could fill a book! The reality is that it is how you feel that is important. If you feel that it was traumatic, then it was. If you dismiss how it is making you feel, trying to put on a brave face to everyone around you, it will be hard to heal. As we said before just as a physical wound needs to be acknowledged, treated and cared for, when a traumatic birth leaves an emotional wound it needs to be acknowledged, treated and cared for too. There are no worse births, only your birth and how it made you feel.

Yes, comparing is human nature but when it comes to trauma it can be damaging. Instead, find your truth, and understand your reality and what that means to you.

Do not berate yourself for how you feel.

There wasn't a day that went by when I didn't berate myself for how I felt. It didn't matter what emotion it was I would beat myself with it.

How you feel matters because your emotions are trying to tell you something. They tell you when something is good for you, they also tell you when you need to address something. Instead of listening to them and then looking at what they mean, you can instead go one of two ways. You can become numb, detaching from the emotions that your experience is causing because you find them so overwhelming. Or you may instead berate yourself for them and do everything to make them go away. This is something we will look at in a later chapter, but it is enough to say at this point that part of healing is acceptance of the emotions you feel and then understanding why you feel that way.

This applies too when it comes to letting others dismiss your experience. Sadly, it is not uncommon for those around you to try to minimise your experience. Sometimes this is done out of concern for you as they seek to make you feel less upset by what has happened or to encourage you to try to feel better or forget it. Of course, they do this out of love and because they just want you to be ok. However, this can mean that because you have no safe place to voice how you feel you can instead feel silenced. This can then result in you berating yourself more as you try to please others by burying your true feelings. Again this is not helpful to healing.

This was a particularly difficult part of my trauma in that I felt like no one would acknowledge what I had been through. Every time I tried to talk about my birth I would be shushed, told not to think about it or told that I needed to just concentrate now on my baby. I couldn't however just ignore what had happened, I had so much that I didn't understand, blank parts in my memory, things that I could not explain, and I felt that no one cared. Instead, everyone's expectation of me was to move on. So, when the feelings were overwhelming me I would become frustrated with myself. In time this led to feeling isolated and alone, lost like I was carrying a huge weight, with no end in sight. I began to try and deny my feelings, deny my experience. I even began to blame myself that I was weak and yes, comparing myself to other women and berating myself believing that I should be able to just get past it. It became a battle that I fought every day, but it was a battle that I would not be able to win until my experience had the acknowledgement it needed.

Trauma isn't something that just goes away. It is carried with you until it is supported to heal. Yes for trauma to heal it also needs to be acknowledged. While our experience cannot be changed, if it is acknowledged it can allow for the gaining of insight into what you need to heal. When there is acceptance of your experience, an understanding of it and an awareness of how it is impacting you, it allows for reflection on how to move beyond it and find ways to find peace again.

Exploring your Experience

What can help with healing is to gently explore, when you're ready, your birth experience.

You can do this by yourself or with someone you trust. The point is to have a safe space to allow you to explore your experience. This is not to relive the trauma, reliving the trauma can cause more hurt and damage, but rather it involves exploring what happened in the sense of how it made you feel and the sensations this evokes. This then allows you to gain an awareness of what you need to heal, such as mourning the things you lost or the changes associated with your birth experience. It is also about providing a safe space to grieve that this wasn't how you thought your birth would be.

It can be incredibly healing to be heard, to not be judged but instead have the safety of sharing your birth experience knowing that your feelings matter and so do you. Even if you decide to do this alone, creating a safe place for yourself emotionally where you do not judge yourself, berate yourself or compare yourself with others, can be liberating. Spending time understanding what your experience has meant to you, allows you then to look at healing.

Trying to silence your trauma leads to the death of your emotional soul. You may think that you can control your pain, your fear and other emotions by silencing it but it will only grow stronger. Yet when you give your experience the space it needs, you allow for something to happen, you take back control. When you say what hurt you, when you say what was done to you, and when this is met by being listened to and understood, it changes how you understand the trauma itself. It also means learning to be honest about your experience even if that truth is painful.

So, exploring your experience will be hard because it means owning your birth. It also means reflecting on an experience that has been very difficult and will bring up uncomfortable feelings for you. This part of the process while difficult, can also allow you to understand better, things you hadn't before considered. This was true for me.

It took a long time for me to understand my experience, I found that especially at night I would struggle, this was when my panic attacks always happened and when I felt most anxious. Over time I reflected that when I was in hospital it was the night-times that held me in terror. This was often when my care was most neglected, where I felt most alone and vulnerable. It was at night that the cries of other babies surrounded me, loudly piercing the still of night as I longed for my daughter who lay what felt like a million miles away in neonatal. My association with the night wasn't a good one, and my brain remembered. It was seeking to keep me safe because for me night-time had become a fearful place where I was in anguish and pain, left feeling alone and scared.

Once I knew this, I could begin to change how my experience had affected me. I needed to feel safe at night again and this was something I could control and actively do. I couldn't change what had happened those long nights in the hospital, but the pain and fear night-time now brought to me, I could change. Little by little I made steps to make night-time safe again, to help my brain see I was safe, that I was no longer in that hospital room but instead safe, and surrounded by people that loved me.

When I started to see where I could make changes it empowered me and also made me realise that I was stronger than I thought, and it carried me through. I saw that I needed to be kinder to myself and accept that I did all I could in circumstances that I had no control over. That I hadn't failed my daughter, but rather that I had fought with all my might to be there for her. Sometimes reflection allows for a change in our focus and a change in our perspective from the trauma lens.

Time may be needed as you revisit painful memories to process the emotions that they incite. If you find that the emotions are overwhelming take a break and ground yourself back to now, using distraction, deep breathing and calming thoughts. You can return at another time to look again at the memories. Sometimes it can be helpful to view your memories as a bystander, like a story playing out of which you are an observer. It can also be helpful to remember that any uncomfortable bodily reactions you may feel are temporary and this in turn can help you to tolerate them, thus losing your fear of them. With time you can see the association between these uncomfortable sensations and your thoughts. This awareness allows you to safely explore your experience without causing more distress, while adjusting your perception of it and thus processing it, allowing you to heal.

It may be that you have gaps in your memory or questions that you need to be answered from your birth experience. This can be supported by a debrief at the hospital where you had your baby. A debrief is usually with a doctor or a midwife and is offered so you can discuss your medical notes and ask any questions that you have. It is important though that you feel ready to explore your medical notes and hear the answers they may contain, and it is good to remember also that sometimes a debrief can focus on just the medical side of your experience and not acknowledge the emotional impact on you. Especially as hearing what happened or learning information that you did not know can be hard. A debrief can be helpful to provide the answers to what happened and why, again this can give space for reflection or a change in focus or understanding of the events.

For me once I explored and owned my experience, accepting that I had been through a very traumatic time and that being expected to just ignore it or move on from it was not helping me to heal, I felt a peace return. I realised that just like any other trauma a person may go through, it leaves its mark, and time plus the right support is needed to heal. It meant that I could be honest with myself and others about how it had impacted me and also being a mother to my daughter. I also saw that instead of trying to bury deep inside me all my pain I could embrace it, mourn it, grieve it and accept it. Accepting and owning my experience was to say that I had done the best I could in the circumstances I found myself in, with the knowledge that I had at that time. That I had in many ways been let down by those in place to care for me and it was unrealistic for me, or anyone around me, to think that none of it mattered. It did matter because I mattered.

Over the years I have seen the impact of women owning their experience. I have seen them go from being in pain to understanding what happened and taking back control. I have seen them grieve what they lost, let go of guilt and dampen down anger. I have seen them realise that they did not have to compare themselves to others but see their ability to accept their experience and in turn, with time, see a different perspective and even find peace.

Your birth, what you went through, what you survived, what that experience means to you, as well as what you do know, but also what you did not know, are so important. When you explore your narrative, it helps you to process your experience and helps you make sense of it. So often birth trauma is a feeling of a loss of control, but by exploring your experience you choose to take that control back.

Exploring and owning your experience is a step to healing. It means knowing that you deserve to be heard and that all you have gone through needs to be acknowledged. When you embrace your experience, you can then use it as a foundation to build on, to help you seek the support you need and begin your journey to a better future. Your experience is yours alone and by taking the time to see what that means for you, it will enable you to heal beyond birth trauma.

A reflection for you.

Sharing my story helped me heal so much. It was hard to see written in words what I had endured, but somehow it enabled me to make sense of it and also challenge my perception of it. We can dismiss our experience or try to minimise it, often because we cannot believe it to be true, but exploring our story can be powerful and healing.

'From times of old the telling of our story has been regarded as a gift and in return the gift it may give you, is to heal.'

- Allow yourself to explore how you feel about your birth experience. Do not deny or try to fight how you feel. Be honest with yourself and be accepting of it. Write down the thoughts and feelings that come to mind and let them pour from your heart as if writing to yourself. Do not think about anyone else, only about what your experience means to you. What are the things you wish were different? What things did you lose that were important to you? Why did this matter to you?
- Then pay attention to how you would feel if this were a friend's notes that you were reading, what would you want them to know? Let your heart fill with compassion for the pain and emotions behind the words. This is the compassion you need to show yourself as you own your experience and seek to heal beyond birth trauma.

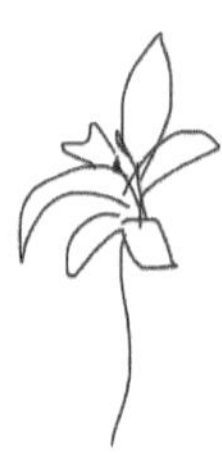

GROUNDING YOURSELF

Earlier in this chapter I mentioned using grounding techniques for times when you feel overwhelmed or disconnected due to the emotions that may visit you while exploring your birth experience. There are many grounding techniques, find the one that works for you.

Here are two that I use.

Listen to your surroundings.

When troublesome thoughts threatened to steal my inner peace I would look to nature to bring relief. I would close my eyes and let my senses tune into the world around me. The warmth of the sun on my face, birds singing nearby. The smell of the trees in the breeze or the scent of beautiful flowers. Sometimes it was the excited voices of my daughters as they played, or the sound of faraway people busy in their day. I would let the sound wash over me, remind me of the here and now. Remind me that I was safe and to find calm. Try this too, let nature be a source of healing.

A cup of tea and a belly laugh.

I always think that there isn't much in life that can't be made better by a good cup of tea and a good laugh. So when I felt overwhelmed with difficult emotions on would go the kettle and I would find something to make me laugh even though it was the last thing I felt like doing. Sometimes it would be funny cat videos, a favourite movie clip or a funny joke I had heard many times before. Or I would tickle my daughters and let their infectious giggles warm my tired soul. The warm feeling of laughter would ease through my body and chase away the murmurs of painful memories. Try it, let laughter be a source of healing.

y

6

Y - YOU MATTER

"I wish I could show you when you are lonely or in darkness, the astonishing light of your own being."
Rumi

"Everyone kept telling me that I had a healthy baby and I had to focus on her, no one seemed to see me, I felt invisible like I just didn't matter."
Claire

A healthy baby isn't all that matters, it is important that you also are healthy both physically and emotionally. You are both linked by every cell in your body, a dyad each as important and equal in needing to be cared for as the other. So much of the focus after birth is on the new baby and of course, this is understandable. Sometimes though you may feel that your own well-being has taken a back seat, that how you are doing is less important than your baby's needs, but this is just not true. Mothers and babies matter equally and your baby's well-being is linked to your own.

After a difficult birth, the impact on you both can be profound. While much care may be given to your baby especially if they have been born early or sick it matters that your well-being is also taken into account and you are able to get the help and support you need, both in a physical sense, but emotionally too. You need to be nurtured, so in turn, you can nurture your baby. It is often the case however that while you may find your baby's well-being is checked with many assessments, with healthcare professionals enquiring about all aspects of your baby's needs your own emotional well-being is left unnoticed, even neglected.

Being a parent let's be honest is hard, not only physically with the sleepless nights and a little human that needs you every second of every day, but emotionally too. Navigating parenthood while making sure you are emotionally ok is challenging, to say the least. Taking care of your physical needs can itself be a major event, it can be halfway through the day and you still haven't managed to get dressed or find the time to eat, so to also think about protecting your emotional well-being can feel impossible. Add to this a traumatic birth, feelings that you do not understand or are overwhelming, and your emotional health can take a massive hit.

It can be hard to voice that you are struggling in your new role as a parent. Fear of what may happen, or that you may be judged as to your parenting, can stop you from telling anyone or reaching out for support. With such a massive change to your life, you can feel like you just don't matter, that your identity, who you were before is lost as you try to navigate your new responsibilities. Fading into the background you can start to feel invisible, life is taken over by this tiny person who needs you and is now your whole life.

Many worry too about saying they are finding being a new parent hard for fear that this will be viewed as not loving their baby, or that it means they are a bad parent. The pressure to be ok, to be an Instagram family, to have everything together and to be back to normal can be overwhelming. So, is it any wonder that many will voice they feel that their emotional health suffers as a result? A difficult birth can compound this and can leave you feeling like you have been permanently changed, and that you don't know yourself anymore.

As you attempt to manage the demands of being a new parent but also the impact a difficult birth has had, the future can start to seem bleak.

After my daughter's birth, she needed to be cared for in the neonatal unit. We spent five weeks in the unit and the focus was on her well-being and needs. Health-wise, feeding, weight gain, blood sugars so much to make sure she was ok and thriving. This of course was needed after all she was premature, and making sure that she was healthy enough to come home was the main priority. However, I felt like I just didn't exist. I felt in the way most of the time especially being still so unwell as I tried to shuffle around the tiny room on the unit in my wheelchair. I don't remember ever being asked how I was or how I was coping in the aftermath of her birth, as I tried to heal from the physical injuries and complications.

The neonatal unit was scary, my tiny daughter in a plastic box, wires everywhere, machines beeping and alarms sounding. I was terrified to touch her, so I would sit and stare at her tiny face for hours. The constant sound of the alarms, the fear that she would take a turn for the worse or that she may not survive at all left me anxious and on high alert. This was my life for weeks and I soon felt I had been on the unit for what seemed like an eternity. I felt almost like the world outside no longer existed, I slept in a chair by her bed and ate in the tiny parent's room at the end of the unit. I had no concept of time, whether it was sunny outside or pouring down with rain. My world had shrunk and it took a toll on me emotionally.

Being on the unit every day meant I didn't see my midwife for any postnatal checks either physically or mentally. My body was still ravaged by birth, but I had no time to notice or care for myself because my tiny daughter lay fighting to survive and this was all that consumed me. This came at the expense of my own wellbeing especially emotionally. I felt on autopilot wading through each day, hoping that one day we would be able to go home.

Once we did go home again the emphasis was on my daughter, whether was she growing, and was her development ok, everything felt like a constant checklist, like I was being assessed on my competency to care for her. No one had prepared me for life with a premature baby and it was terrifying. I was used to having the neonatal staff there to call on at any moment but now I was all alone. Fear and anxiety escalated and my mental health was declining as I felt the weight of such a huge responsibility.

While everyone was concerned about my daughter, I felt alone and invisible and consumed with anxiety yet strove even more to wear the mask of being ok. Even when I did try to voice how I was feeling my cries for help were dismissed, and my anguish was ignored, so I would fall silent again and try to carry on.

As the months went by and I was still struggling I didn't know where to turn. My daughter was doing really well and no longer a cause for concern. Yet for me, it was a different story, birth trauma had left its mark and was tainting everything. I always describe it as if my trauma was like a poison that was slowly running through my veins, seeping into every aspect of my world, slowly draining me of life, of hope.

Not expecting too much of You!

While it can be easy to neglect your own needs with a family to care for, part of healing, especially after a difficult birth is acknowledging that your well-being matters. That you also need and deserve love, care, support and help. How can you support your healing and show that you matter too?

As new parents you can expect yourself to be able to continue life as it was before, able to do everything while also being there for everyone else, including your new baby and this can be emotionally draining. As a result, you can find that you push your physical and emotional needs to the side, residing at the bottom of a very long list. After pregnancy and birth a period of transition and recovery is needed especially to recover from a traumatic birth which requires you to take time to heal and access the right support.

It is important that you make time for yourself to be physically cared for by rest, the right nutrition and protecting your emotional health. You also need to be realistic about what you can and can't do. This is hard and I have found most new parents will struggle with this, but you mustn't overload yourself and make yourself even more mentally or physically exhausted.

Asking and accepting help will give you the support you need to recover. Don't be afraid to ask those around you to help out in practical ways. Again this can be hard if you are used to just getting on with things, and not needing anyone. Realising that your well-being takes priority over the things you normally do can be a challenge, it requires you to 'let go' and allow things to give a little. This may go against the grain especially if you are a very organised and orderly person, like me.

It means acknowledging that you are healing and as such it means being kinder to yourself and what you expect of yourself. This was something I especially struggled with. I liked order, and a neat, clean home, it was something I had no issues maintaining before I had my daughter. Yet after her birth, I found this overwhelming and also that my own needs were always lost in the demands of daily life. I could never ask for help but instead struggled on despite some days being virtually on my knees with exhaustion. Physically I would push myself beyond what was reasonable, especially in the early weeks and months when my body was still trying to recover from the birth. I'm ashamed to say that I neglected myself and in doing so this went against my desire to heal.

I always talk to parents about how when they travel on an aeroplane the flight attendant will run through the advice about what to do in an emergency. The advice is always that should oxygen be needed from the overhead masks they are to put their masks on first and then help others. Of course, this isn't human nature we often rush to help others at the expense of ourselves, but to steal a well-known phrase, we cannot pour from an empty cup! The reality is that before we can care for others we first must care for ourselves. As mothers especially we often find ourselves at the bottom of a very long list of things that need our attention, to the detriment of ourselves.

Another aspect of expecting too much is having such high expectations of yourself that you forget to see and celebrate, the things that you have achieved each day. It may be just getting out of bed and surviving the day, which on some days will be all you can manage. You can become so fixated on the long list of things that you believe you must achieve that you set yourself up for failure every day.

Shifting your focus allows you to see what you are achieving, as opposed to what you think you should be achieving. Being realistic and being aware that you are on a journey of healing will keep you from demanding too much of yourself. It will allow you instead to realise that life has changed and as such this means caring for a new baby as well as trying to recover physically and emotionally from a difficult birth requires a consideration of what is realistic.

Consideration of your emotional needs will also mean the need to put in place healthy boundaries. Boundaries are things that you decide are helpful to protect you emotionally and usually involve your relationships with others. This can be hard with those you love, but it is important so they do not set unrealistic expectations or demands on you that don't allow you the time to reflect and find the support you need to heal. This can be challenging as they may find these new boundaries unfamiliar and may push against them. An example of a healthy boundary is reviewing what you are able to do for others now you have the responsibility of a new baby. Knowing you matter and putting in place boundaries that support you shows that you are starting to walk your road to healing.

I remember years ago seeing a woman at home who was struggling after a difficult birth. As I looked at her across the room, her eyes were sunken and heavy, her skin was pale and what struck me most was how hunched over she was, like a tiny animal that was seeking to curl up in a ball to protect itself. As we talked she explained to me how the two days before she had spent many hours making food for a family gathering that weekend. Rising early morning and going to bed late at night, all while trying to care for her newborn. We explored together how this expectation of what she believed she needed to do, including making others happy, was actually unrealistic and was instead making her physically exhausted and emotionally too. It almost felt like she was imploring me for permission to rest, and during our time together I helped her to reflect that the permission she needed came from herself. This included advocating for herself and her needs and also asking for help.

Yes the demands we put on ourselves or allow others to put on us can be heavy, these can be a lot to carry on the challenging road to healing. What can help you to lighten this load, to help you continue to find the way ahead?

Time

Time does not magically heal the hurt or take away the pain of a difficult birth but time does allow you the chance to process your feelings, reach out for help and find what you need to heal. There is no time limit on healing, it will take as long as it takes. You must however make time and space to do what is needed to heal and this can be a difficult barrier to navigate. This includes allowing time to give attention and tend to your own needs.

A self-care plan can support you with this. A self-care plan may include things that help you to feel calm, support physical well-being or help you to feel positive about yourself and the world around you, or are practical to manage the demands of family life. For me, this includes immersing myself in nature. I love being out in the fresh air, it helps me to feel free and distracted from the worries that may cloud my mind. A walk in the bright sun or even on a rainy day helps clear my mind. It reminds me that beauty is all around me, that the world is so much bigger than what is consuming me and it grounds me to the present, even when my mind seeks to drag me elsewhere. This was something I did once we were both home from the hospital. I would pop my daughter in the pram and go for a walk.

Realising you matter and putting in place ways to support this is a firm foundation on which healing can begin. Find time to look for ways to start building this foundation. This is very individual, and you are the best person to know what is right for you. It may then help to sit with those close to you and talk through what you need to help you as you heal. This may be practical support or emotional support. Communication with those you love is vital as it means that they are able to understand better what you need.

It has been said to me many times that finding time to care for yourself with a new baby to look after is hard. I am not going to disagree, it is hard. However, if you are reading this book then I know you are at the place where you want to start your journey to healing, and as I said at the start the road is hard. There are no shortcuts, I wish there were as I would happily show you the way and guide you to it. Some of that road will involve hard work and this is so true when it comes to finding time for your emotional well-being. It may go against the grain for you, you may even feel selfish after all, it may have been a long time since you thought about what you needed. As the beginning of the chapter said, you and your baby both deserve to have your needs met. Not doing so is detrimental to you both. Start small, every small step matters on your road.

Time will be affected too by other circumstances and outside influences. You may find that others will try to encroach on the time you set aside to heal. It can help if you explain to them how important it is to you and your journey of healing and how you need their support. This ties in with the healthy boundaries that we mentioned above.

If time is being taken up by busy family life, try to sit down as a family and see where you can make changes that can allow for your needs to be supported. As a couple, you have just been through a life-changing event, life is not the same as it was before your baby arrived. Time to reflect on what has changed and what adaptions need to be made to support you both can draw you closer and help you manage your new family life.

Each stage of your healing will also take different amounts of time. You may find that understanding what happened to you medically is quicker to process, but the effect on you and your life emotionally may take much longer. It doesn't matter what time is needed for each stage because we all process things very differently, we all heal differently. Whatever the case be kind to yourself, do not expect too much and allow time to navigate your road to healing.

Rest

Getting adequate rest is important. Especially while healing being able to rest matters. This means looking at ways to make this possible within your family circumstances. It may mean again asking others for help or letting the house go un-hoovered. It may mean looking for ways to have small amounts of time to yourself or adjusting the family schedule to allow for some downtime. Rest will also be different for each person. Rest may be actual sleep, or it may be doing an activity you enjoy. It may be time to chat with a friend, going for a walk, a cuddle on the sofa with your little one or even just a cup of tea and a nice piece of cake. The point is it doesn't matter what you do to rest, only that you do it.

It is believed that there is a link between sleep and how we process memories and experiences, as such making sure you are getting adequate rest and sleep is important. Trauma affects the way you process experiences and memories, and often rest is therefore impacted. Being able to rest is just as important as making sure you are watered and fed.

Getting sleep with a new baby is difficult, to say the least, so finding other ways to rest your mind can help while healing. Nightmares may break your sleep or unwanted memories may keep you tossing and turning until morning light. So rest is not just about sleeping but ways that allow your mind to rest from the thoughts that seek to fill, even torment it.

There are many good apps that you can find for your phone that can allow you to practice relaxation and deep breathing exercises which can be helpful to bring calm. If this isn't for you then find other ways that allow your mind to rest. Reading can be helpful, as can anything else that distracts you from troublesome thoughts. As I mentioned I love to take my camera and go out to capture the beauty of nature. For others, it may be physical activity or time with friends or family. Just a few hours of mindful rest can work wonders to restore a tired soul.

One of the times I cherished, when I found I could rest my mind, was when I was breastfeeding my daughter. It was the only time that I was sat down and unable to do anything else. This was when I felt my most calm and I would just sit and look at her, stroking her golden hair and wondered how I had created something so amazing. Sometimes you can be so consumed with all the things you seem to need to get done that you forget to stop and just take in that moment in time. This is where mindfulness can be helpful. Mindfulness is just that being mindful of where you are now. It allows you to come back from the things in the past that have hurt you or from future worries that can overwhelm you to the moment that is here right now, this can be where rest can be found. It can be said that a lot of anxiety is about the past or the future, so being able even for a few moments to reside in the present can give a little space from the worries that devour your mind.

Resting will help your mind to again find moments of peace and calm. Life can be chaotic and a merry-go-round that never seems to stop, this can hinder you on your road to healing, seeking to divert you on paths that take you away from your much-desired destination. There can be no time to see that you matter too.

Rest and time out from the constant demands of life are vital to helping you refocus so you can see more clearly the road ahead to healing.

Physical Healing

Birth trauma takes a physical toll on your body. After nine months of nurturing and growing your baby and then the birth itself, physically even after a positive birth experience, it takes time to heal. When birth is difficult, or complicated by medical interventions, severe blood loss or physical damage the time needed to recover can be days, weeks or even months. You can be tempted to try to return to normal trying to spring back to how you were before your birth, while also trying to cope with how you have been affected and do everything that you or others expect of you. It is important however that you allow yourself time to heal physically.

Physical health and emotional health are just as important as each other and are linked in so many ways. For us to heal emotionally, we must also heal physically. The road to healing involves not only healing emotionally but physically too. Neglecting either will serve to stumble your journey.

This was something that I personally had to confront. The severe blood loss and resulting anaemia I experienced left me with a long recovery for many months. I also had damage to some of my organs from the pre-eclampsia that required management and time to heal. It meant that physically I was very weak, prone to infections and unable to do what I had previously. I also had severe physical scars from the surgery to remove my placenta that required careful care. I often felt very down with my limitations, I had gone from being a fit and healthy young woman to convalescing. Many times, I would try to do too much and push myself beyond my physical abilities to the detriment of myself not only physically, but emotionally too. My body was a wreck and it was trying to tell me that it needed time to heal. In reality, it took a good year to recover and heal physically from my birth.

When the physical damage suffered at birth is long-lasting, it is important that you get the help and treatment you need for any medical needs to be managed. This can be hard when feeling traumatised and emotionally scarred. Even the thought of any medical treatment can be terrifying and lead to feelings of panic. Getting the needed treatment is an important part of your healing and you may need specialist support emotionally for you to manage this part of your journey. Trust in healthcare providers may have been broken and it can be hard to place trust in them again. It is vital that you communicate with them how you have been affected and the support you need to get the medical help you require. Ask someone to advocate for you if you find this hard such as your partner or close friend/family member.

Also, do not allow yourself to be dismissed if you do seek help for your physical recovery. Sadly when it comes to women's gynaecological health finding someone who will listen to your symptoms can be hard. If you are still experiencing difficulties from the birth of your baby talk to a doctor who will understand and offer the treatment you need. I have known women to struggle for many years with the physical issues of a difficult birth.

Physical well-being cannot be something you neglect, it also needs your time and attention. You matter, as a whole. Both the physical you, as well as the emotional you.

Learn about Trauma

Knowledge is power they say and learning about trauma can be your secret weapon. Learning about how it happens, how it changes the brain and what the effects of trauma are can help you see that trauma is a result of what has happened to you and doesn't have anything to do with you as a person.

Trauma can eat away at your sense of self-belief, your self-esteem, your personal identity and your purpose in life. You can feel like you will never be ok again and that you don't know yourself anymore. This can mean you not seeing how you matter both to those around you and also to the world in general. You can lose sight of your self-worth as you see each day as a battle you're not sure you can face. Sadly for some, this can lead to feelings that others would be better off without them or that they are a burden to those they love.

When you learn about trauma you will see that your trauma didn't happen because you are weak, or because you were not prepared. Your trauma wasn't because you did anything wrong or because you allowed it to happen. Your trauma happened because your mind was overwhelmed by the distressing, scary, stressful event that was the birth of your baby. Trauma is defined by the experience of the person, meaning it is individual to you.

Understanding trauma can help you make sense of your feelings as well as any physical effects you may suffer.

It will help you to understand that the reason why you are struggling and are full of the difficult emotions you carry each day is because you have been through a traumatic event. Just like you would understand why someone who has been involved in a natural disaster or a violent crime would be affected by their experience, when you understand trauma you can understand why you have been affected by your experience too.

I found that this knowledge was so powerful for me and finally, things began to make sense. I found that the emotions and physical responses I was experiencing suddenly had a reason. This alone took away some of the fear. I wasn't going mad or losing control. I wasn't just unable to cope with life, no, I was traumatised, and I needed help to heal.

Part of knowing that you matter is arming yourself with as much information as you can about trauma and what you will need to move ahead on your road to healing. Many wonderful books explore trauma and its impact, written by individuals who truly understand it. Once I started to understand trauma it started to lose its power over me and I knew I could overcome it. It was no longer a scary unknown monster but a very normal, human reaction to what had happened to me. So use the powerful tool of knowledge to help you navigate the road to healing.

Find Support with Others

For me, a big part of my healing from birth trauma was finding others who had experienced and suffered from it too. To speak to others who understood my feelings, worries and anxieties brought me great solace. I no longer felt alone but wrapped in arms of comfort. I realised that it wasn't just me, that I wasn't weird or strange but that others also had felt as I did and could offer me the support I needed.

Having others around me who had travelled the road to healing gave me the hope I desperately needed to keep going. At times they just took my hand and other times they carried me, as I did for them too.

When we are scared and full of fear, nothing calms us like the reassuring words or loving embrace of someone we trust. Healing comes from gaining a sense of safety, our attachment to others is our greatest defence when we feel at threat. When we connect with others who truly understand it provides emotional safety and empathy for any feelings we may carry of shame, guilt or grief. Building trust again is important, as is finding others to help us manage our fears through their gentle reassurance from having been there too.

Unresolved trauma can take a huge toll on your relationships, so healing matters. Yet being hurt and having your trust broken can mean this is a challenge. Find others that you can trust enough to accompany you on your road to healing, who can safely listen and hold your feelings while helping you find what you need. Let them be like an anchor that holds you steady in the turbulent waves of trauma, seeing the raw, vulnerable, fragile you that you have hidden for so long. This may be your partner, friend or therapist. It doesn't matter who, only that they listen from the heart.

So, seek out others who are healing. You will find that they will be at different stages to you in their journey. This doesn't matter, look to them and draw on their strength to help get you through, knowing that you will be helping them too.

Find What Works For YOU

As you travel towards healing there will be stops along the way that will claim to help and support you. It may be counselling, or other therapies, it may be a de-brief or birth reflection session or peer support, or it may be holistic options such as mindfulness. Whatever is available you need to find what works, for *you*.

Everyone is different, and not every option will be right for you. Some you try will help, and others will knock you back. Whenever I tried something, and it didn't help I would become disillusioned and wonder what was wrong with me. Of course, there was nothing wrong with me I just needed to find what worked for me.

Whenever you find that something does work use it to make you stronger. There's no right or wrong because everyone is unique. Your 'right' of practising mindfulness may be someone else's 'wrong'. So, look around, stop and test things out, if it doesn't feel right move on till you find what works for you. So too with the many therapies that you may be offered. If they don't work don't become discouraged, instead know that healing is just as individual as you are and so finding the right help as you navigate your road will take time.

This book is my journey, and the things that helped and supported me and I hope that they may help you too. They are not however written in stone, but words on paper that can be embraced or erased, rewritten or ignored. Finding your personal healing journey is what matters. Part of that journey however will be you have finally seen that you matter and this is the place where healing can begin to flourish as you start to heal beyond birth trauma.

A reflection for you.

For many years I struggled with believing that because of my birth trauma, I was a burden to everyone around me. My mind would trick me into believing that I didn't matter, and I would imagine how life would be without trauma to taint it and it would break more pieces of my already fragile heart. Yet I was missing something very important. I had lost sight of the fact that I was deeply loved, that it wasn't my fault but that this had been forced upon me and that I was fighting with all my might to heal. Also that I did matter, to my daughters and my family and friends, and that there was so much good surrounding me. I just needed to see it.

What can you do to help you reflect on how much you matter?

- Every day before you close your eyes to sleep think of one special moment that day. It may have been your little one smiling. It may be that you built a tower of blocks or sang a nursery rhyme together, maybe you just held your little one close while they drifted off to sleep. Maybe you achieved something at home or work or showed some kindness to a stranger. Whatever it is, whatever that small moment means to you let it fill your mind and drift to your heart, let it show you all the good that surrounds you and let it whisper, *you matter!*
- Ask loved ones and friends to write you a little note that describes one thing that they love about you. Read these one at a time and take time to reflect on why you matter to those around you, embrace the love they feel for you and see your true worth. Pin these notes up around your home to remind you how much you matter. In the darkest of times, this can help show you the 'astonishing light of your own being'.

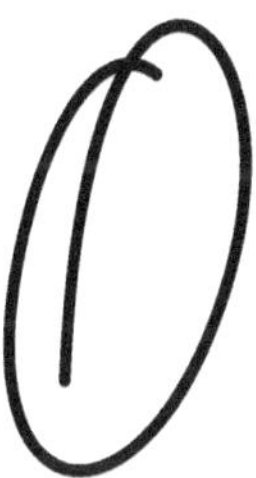

7

O - OPEN TO YOUR EMOTIONS

"You gain strength, courage and confidence by every experience in which you stop and look fear in the face."
Eleanor Roosevelt

"Sometimes the emotions would be so overwhelming that I just wanted to disappear."
Emily

I can feel the tears stinging my eyes. I blink them away and try to let my logical mind silence the thunderous beating in my chest. I look at my daughter, she is smiling, laughing and happy. Guilt stabs at my heart. The what-ifs linger in my mind. Did I do enough to protect her, to keep her safe? Guilt whispers to me increasing the pounding of my heart. Emotions feel so strong, so raw, so many, that it feels like they will overwhelm me. Then the sadness arrives.

Birth trauma is much more than the story of what happened to you. It is the way it has affected you on the inside. Birth trauma robs you of so much, including a feeling of being in control of yourself. Strong emotions can take over making you feel overwhelmed, these can then be felt in very physical ways. This can be a scary part of birth trauma, causing you to feel you have lost yourself, or even that you are losing your mind.

As you walk your road to healing you will need to find yourself again, this includes being open to the emotions that you may be feeling as a result of your birth experience. This can be one of the hardest parts of healing beyond birth trauma because your emotions will be many and varied, they are also very strong and as a result evoke very real, physical responses.

The emotions and accompanying physical sensations that you experience during your birth are remembered, and your brain makes strong connections between what happened and the way it made you feel. After the event not only will you have memories of what happened but also experience very real physical reactions to those memories. Think for a moment of a happy time you had, perhaps with a loved one and notice the emotions you feel, connection, laughter, happiness and contentment. Now think about a time when you watched a scary movie, what emotions does this bring back to you?

The emotional part of your brain expresses itself in very physical ways. When you are scared it is usually a pounding heart, nausea or fast breathing, crying and the urge to protect yourself. In the case of birth trauma, your mind and body store the emotions that it felt at the time such as fear, but then also the physical reactions you experienced related to that emotion such as panic. As a result, even though the events have now passed any time you remember or are reminded of anything related to the birth it may evoke those very strong emotions and the physical reactions that it made the connection with. Your natural response, therefore, is to avoid anything that makes you feel both the emotion and the strong physical reaction, as these often can be a cause of great distress.

It is not just memories that can cause such strong physical reactions, the brain loves to make other connections and meaning out of things you experience. Mostly this is a good thing like happy memories of blissful holidays but in the case of birth trauma, the brain can make connections with things that normally would be ok and safe instead to something that feels dangerous and distressing. After a difficult birth, this can be anything related to pregnancy or birth, situations that involve anything medical. It may be TV shows that show pregnancy or birth or contain threat or suspense. It may be anything related to your health or that of your baby. Even just going out into a world that you may now feel is unsafe. Some women find even their own baby to be a source of distress, a reminder of the awful things they experienced, this can be especially distressing. These connections in turn then result in very real physical reactions that can leave you reeling, feeling out of control and full of fear and anxiety.

The emotions and the physical reactions they evoke can be so overwhelming that you can try to feel nothing, attempting to numb and block your emotions for fear they may open a floodgate you fear you cannot stop. You may seek ways to bury your emotions deep within you or even deny them altogether, desperate for them to go away. You may feel shut down as your body, still in survival mode, seeks to protect itself. It is as if a part of you has become fractured, and broken. Trauma becomes stuck in our bodies so to speak, causing all these emotions and physical reactions that are hard to manage, it is as if it cannot complete or release itself.

Trying to manage these emotions and physical reactions requires a lot of energy, and this carries a high price. It can rob you of a loving relationship with yourself, both your body and your mind. Emotions can become like stones that weigh you down, as you try to carry them around every day, becoming so heavy you feel constantly tired making healing beyond birth trauma difficult. While you may seek to banish unwanted emotions, they may still manifest themselves in strong physical reactions, your brain remembers even if you try not to!

Feeling anxious or on edge, agitated or as if on high alert can become a daily companion. This can leave you feeling both physically and emotionally exhausted.

So when it comes to emotions and how they make you feel, it can be hard to explore them because of the strong sensations that accompany them. Yet working through the emotions you have about your birth experience is helpful to healing. Healing doesn't mean that you no longer have any of the unwelcome emotions, but rather that you can experience the memories, the emotions and the physical reactions but that they no longer overwhelm you. Part of this we discussed in chapter three around exploring your experience. This can be the last thing you want to do, again because the emotion and then physical response it evokes can be just too much.

Finding ways that help you to understand the emotion you are experiencing and then how you can cope with the physical response is part of the healing journey. While this does not change what happened, it can help you understand why and how you feel such emotions, and in turn, can give you freedom from the fear that accompanies them, allowing you to feel a sense of safety again.

Restoring balance requires you to have a self-awareness of your emotions, the response you may have to them and how they are linked to your birth experience. The only way you can cope with the emotions that flood you after a traumatic birth is to become aware of your inner turmoil and then befriend it.

Emotions everywhere

When you are traumatised, you can be scared to feel. While your trauma may have passed the emotions are still very much here, often holding you captive, living in fear of both the emotional and the physical sensations that can result. I liken it to a movie reel that is stuck on repeat.

Trauma tries to keep us watching the movie and feeling the emotions too!

Many emotions can accompany birth trauma such as guilt, anguish, anger, grief, sadness, sorrow, loss, fear, hopelessness, blame, frustration or shame. You may have some, or all of these emotions or ones not listed here. Each one is valid. Each emotion matters. Your emotions can collide or change, or you may find they come in stages. You may feel guilt which in turn gives way to anger or vice versa. It may be that anguish gives way to hopelessness. It is also important to say that emotions can co-exist. You can feel frustration while also feeling sadness, blame as well as shame. This applies too for other emotions that are not part of your birth trauma. It is completely possible to be happy that your beautiful baby is here, while also feeling sad about how your baby came into the world.

Emotions give space for reflection

Your emotions are important, they are gateways that serve to provide reflection so you can begin to heal beyond birth trauma. Being open to your emotions allows you to understand why you feel the emotion, how it relates to what you have been through and why it matters to healing. It can bring discomfort but then also relief when it has the space to be understood. This can be explained by the example of guilt.

Guilt is a very common emotion that accompanies birth trauma. There can be so many reasons that you may feel the emotion of guilt. When you are open to the emotion you are feeling you are able to explore the emotion, understand it and see if there is a basis for how you're feeling. This in turn can bring relief. How?

While it will be painful to admit your feeling of guilt, doing so can bring firstly a sense of relief at being able to finally let out how you truly feel. Then, when your feelings of guilt are explored often it can be seen that there was no basis for them and so you can be released from the feeling, which means then peace can be found. What do I mean?

When I think about my journey to healing guilt was something that held me back, a heavy weight that I carried with me for so long. Honestly, I felt guilty about everything and would constantly play over and over in my mind how I could have done things differently. Over the many years I have spent supporting families guilt is the emotion that always seems to scream most loudly to be heard and be the most reluctant to let go.

Guilt can take many forms. Guilt can be feelings of not having done enough or of not in some way having prevented your trauma. It can be over how you did or didn't birth, or if you had a medical intervention. It could be guilt over not having had that instant rush of love for your baby, or not being able to breastfeed. You may think if only you had done this or if only you had known that, then maybe things would have been different again causing feelings of guilt.

Guilt is powerful because along with guilt there is blame. When something bad happens you can look to assign blame as it can discharge the discomfort and help you feel in control. Sadly though you often level that blame at yourself, only amplifying the guilt. I have honestly heard the pain of guilt replayed over and over so many times, and seen the pain that it has caused etched on so many faces.

Yet when you explore emotions such as guilt and seek to understand where they have come from, you can begin to see they are often not based in reality, that there are no bases for self-blame, and that are you instead seeing things through a trauma lens. Let me explain.

For a long time, I believed my birth experience was my fault. It was my fault I was traumatised, that the care I received while giving birth had left me hurt and broken, an empty shell. It was my fault that my body wasn't able to keep my baby safe which meant instead of going home, we became consumed by the journey of neonatal that had left me scared and protective of my tiny daughter. Guilt was making me believe that everything that had happened was because I had caused it. My guilt remained, strong and unyielding. I questioned everything. Did I do anything that caused my pre-eclampsia? Did I cause my placenta to get stuck, or the haemorrhage that nearly took me from this world? Was I difficult to care for? Did I not try hard enough to get well quicker, so I could care for my baby? Was it my fault that I didn't know what was happening to my baby those first few days when I couldn't see her, all the lost moments, the lost time? Guilt was powerful and held on to me and just wouldn't let go. What though was the reality?

My reality was that I had done the best I could in the most awful of circumstances, with events that were out of my control and with the best knowledge I had at that time.

For me, one of the things I felt most guilty about was not being there for my baby in those first hours and days. While she lay what felt like a million miles away in the neonatal unit, I was in the high-dependency unit fighting to stay alive. I remember the staff bringing me this tiny photo of her in an incubator, wires everywhere the first time I saw her since she had been taken from me and all I wanted to do was to be with her. My heart was shattering into pieces but I couldn't be with her, it simply wasn't possible because I needed medical care too. I remember closing my eyes and wishing that it was all just a bad dream, hoping that if I opened them again everything would be ok and she would be here for me to hold and love. Even when I was able to finally visit her my body was so ravaged by the blood loss and surgery that I was too weak to even hold her.

Once we went home I would torment myself about these times, berate myself for not pushing myself more, and visions of her lying all alone in her incubator would wake me at night. I would dream about walking around the hospital trying to find her, calling out her name. My heart was torn by physical pain that I wasn't there when they were endlessly teasing drops of blood from her already bruised feet to test her blood sugars, that I couldn't hold and comfort her. Guilt consumed me and placed its anchor in my soul and I carried it around like a crushing weight.

Hindsight is a wonderful thing and when looking through hindsight-tinted glasses, we see things so different. We need to remember that in times of stress, we go into survival mode, seeking to protect ourselves and those we love. The logical part of our brain is switched off and instead, the very primal part takes over, we go into fight, flight or freeze mode. This means we will do things that later we may struggle to understand. To protect ourselves we may disassociate from what is happening around us, we may lash out fighting as it were to try to escape what is happening. In birth, many will instead freeze like a tiny animal in front of its predator, becoming complicit, giving in, and allowing things to happen to them that they didn't want. Women have said to me that in life they are strong characters, have very responsible careers, and are confident and able to advocate for themselves, yet in the birth room they found themselves without a voice and felt defenceless and vulnerable. Guilt has then set in as to why they became as if tiny prey at the mercy of their experience.

With time I was able to explore my emotion of guilt and see the reality of what was my experience. This in turn provided a release from it and a finding of peace. I wasn't to blame for my trauma, I did the best I could for me and my daughter. I had given everything I could at a time when I was vulnerable and deeply traumatised. My guilt wasn't based in reality, but instead a false reality that birth trauma had created. Being able to see the true reality allowed me to slowly be released from the guilt, self-blame and any physical feelings that accompanied it.

The emotions I felt such as guilt also allowed me to do something else they allowed me to reflect and see they were important and needed. How?

Each emotion serves a purpose in healing. Guilt allowed me to see that it wasn't my fault and that other things had caused my trauma, I could then reduce my inner critic that strove to make me feel I wasn't good enough, or I had failed. Guilt then moved to anger which taught me that I had a right to be angry for the poor care I endured, how it had changed me and all the things I had lost as a result. Anger in turn became grief as I grieved the loss of my birth experience and felt the hurt of how my life had now changed. This then gave way to frustration at the loss of control, and how my birth trauma had affected me and impacted my journey as a mother. Then slowly something happened. I started to feel other emotions too such as the determination to find support and not let what happened define me. Also, courage to start the road to healing. Yes, my emotions while unpleasant served a purpose, I just had to find it. So what about other emotions such as sadness?

Why sadness matters?

So with birth being an event that we usually associate with happiness, what happens if instead of feeling happy you feel sad?

As we have already said all of our emotions are important, including sadness. When it comes to birth we can often feel that sadness is a negative emotion, having no place in our life with the arrival of a new baby and so we seek to turn sadness into what we think we 'should' feel. You may seek to fight your sadness, believing it shows you to have a weakness, or something deflective. You may try to banish the emotion, believing you should just forget and move on, seeking to make yourself feel happy. You may question yourself asking 'Why do I feel this way?', 'What is wrong with me?', or 'Why is everyone else happy but not me?' This can lead to you feeling frustrated.

However your feelings of sadness matter. These feelings tell you that what you have experienced has affected you and as such, needs to be acknowledged and understood. When you fight your sadness, it leaves the feelings raw and not understood. The sadness then can lie within you and lead to other emotions such as hopelessness and even despair. Yet when you open your heart to your feelings of sadness something happens, you allow yourself to understand what your sadness is, why it is here and how you can support it while you heal.

Feeling sad over a birth experience can happen for so many reasons, all of which are valid. If feelings of sadness are there, let them reside with you. Don't fight them but instead explore them. Think about what aspects of your birth experience are causing your sadness. Was it the loss of a wanted experience, the feeling that your choices weren't supported or respected, or maybe feeling a loss of control? Whatever the reasons for your sadness, allow yourself to feel them, and let them be validated and heard.

Part of your journey to healing is not only understanding what is causing your emotion of sadness but also asking yourself how this sadness is manifesting itself. It may be frustration towards others, a quick temper, or being defensive of yourself. Or maybe it is struggling to bond with your new baby, or feeling inadequate as a new parent. Your sadness may be the cause of some reactions that you aren't even aware of.

When you start to understand why you feel sad, it allows you to explore what you need and what will offer you support. This can be very different for each person, indeed for each feeling of sadness. It may be you need a safe place to talk and share your feelings. It may be that you need time to yourself to work through how you feel, and how to manage your feelings. It may be that you need to find answers to the events that happened to help you understand the experience of your birth.

Your sadness, and acknowledgement of it opens space for something else, the showing of yourself kindness, compassion, and even forgiveness. It allows you to see that you lost something that had meaning, that maybe you were a victim of other people's actions or helps you to see you made choices based on the information and circumstances that you had at that time. It allows for self-reflection on what is important to you, what your needs are and how you can seek help to support these. It means a greater understanding of yourself and also what you may need in the future, especially future pregnancies. Fighting your sadness can be stunting to you emotionally and it can trip you up on your road to healing, by letting it reside with you and learning to understand it, it can allow space for healing.

So when you have feelings of sadness accept and acknowledge them and let them reside with you. Investigate the feelings, why they are here and what they can tell you. Allow the feelings to teach you what you need to support yourself. Do not fight them but instead seek to understand your feelings of sadness, embrace them and let them help you to heal. This brings me to another emotion very common after birth trauma, grief.

Grieving the losses

The tears fall staining the front of my dress. Sobs rack my body and I struggle to catch my breath. There is pain deep in my chest, twisting knots that feel like my heart is tearing. This is grief. Grief that needs to be acknowledged and felt.

I have learnt that you cannot run from grief. You need to acknowledge the pain and feel it. It's hard to do and it can take time to walk the path that grief lays before you.

Grief can be like the darkest night, heavy and consuming without light to lead the way. Yet you must pass through the dark until dawn returns because it is part of the healing process as you learn to cope with the things you have been through or lost.

What kind of things can or should you grieve? Birth is not a thing we associate with grief unless of course there is the loss of a baby. You may have planned for a long time the day you bring a baby into the world. Your wishes for that day varied and individual. You made birth plans, attended classes and waited with eager anticipation. Yet if the day arrives and birthing your baby is difficult, thwarted with complications or doesn't happen how you planned, the impact can be profound. You may feel that because your baby is here and all is now perceived to be ok, you should be grateful and that grief has no place in becoming a new parent. Trying to bury feelings that accompany a major change in our lives, however, can lead to us faltering emotionally.

You need to know that it is ok to grieve what was lost. Not having the birth of your baby go as you hoped, even in some cases becoming a traumatic event, needs to be acknowledged. Grieving the loss of an experience you wanted, allowing the emotions that result and having time to feel and process them will allow you to heal beyond it as well as help you find ways to manage the pain.

When birth is traumatic there can be so much that is lost. With my first daughter, I never got those firsts, first cuddles, first feeds, instead, I was separated from her while she lay in the neonatal unit and I lay in the high dependency unit. It bothered me for a long time, ate away at me, inciting guilt and consuming me. Every time I thought about it I had physical pain and I struggled to hold back the tears. What I needed was to let the tears fall and grieve what I had lost. When I finally did this and reflected on my experience, letting the feelings be raw, I felt grief engulf me. What followed in time was as grief was given the space it needed was a deep relief. While I knew I couldn't change the fact that my baby spent her first few days of life without me, I could accept that it wasn't my fault, and I didn't have to pretend this hadn't been hard for me and I could grieve the loss I felt.

In time as my grief began to ease, I was able to finally see other moments that brought light. Despite our separation when I was finally well enough to see my daughter, I put my hand into her incubator and she grasped my finger tight. My first precious moment with her. It wasn't the first cuddles or a first feed, they had been lost but just that tiny grasp was so magical. In embracing my grief, I began to heal the things causing me pain and with that, I found there were other precious memories I could hold on to.

Grieving the loss of a wanted experience that you desired, but didn't happen, matters. Allowing the emotions to be free and feeling them is hard, but also healing. Being able to voice disappointment and loss rather than holding it deep in your heart gives relief. Grieving allows you to see that there is so much that you haven't given yourself credit for.

When you allow feelings to be felt you often find along with the pain, there are also moments of light however fleeting. Giving yourself time to grieve what you wanted but lost isn't wrong but part of taking care of yourself as you walk the road to healing.

It is also important to grieve change. After a difficult birth, your life may look so different and you may struggle to accept this. Not only have things in your life changed but you have changed. You may miss the person you were before. Giving ourselves time to grieve how you and your life have changed isn't wrong but needed to heal.

In time you will find ways to cope with the emotion of grief and sometimes you are even able to find the good. Grieving will be hard, it will mean facing feelings you may have tried to forget. It will take time and support for you to be able to find your way. How you feel matters and never should your feelings be denied the time they need. Allowing grief to sit with you for a while is good because it enables the light to return. You do not have to be brave all the time, you can allow the tears to fall and the pain to be felt. Healing does not mean you forget or pretend that everything is okay. Healing means you find ways to cope, to feel the pain without it overwhelming you and maybe also find memories that bring you a little comfort along the way.

Grief is as important as love, joy and hope. Grief is individual. Grief is just as much a part of our journey as every other emotion we process. Grief is part of what makes us human and grieving loss is what helps us on the road to healing. So be kind to your heart, grieve what you have lost and with that, you will find healing too.

How can you manage difficult emotions?

Your emotions are like a well-tuned orchestra, when working together they are healthy functions that keep you safe, allowing you to experience wonderful things such as falling in love and enabling you to enjoy life. Trauma hijacks your emotions and holds them to ransom. It distorts them and makes you believe that you are losing control or unable to cope with how you feel. This causes you to see the world through traumas distorted lens, including how you view yourself. It is your emotions that are most hurt by trauma and this includes the most sensitive parts that make you loving, creative and imaginative. It causes you to doubt your abilities, causes you to lose trust in the world and those around you and trauma breeds fear.

As humans, we seek connection but the emotions of trauma often mean isolation. Trauma can cause you to do and say things that you wouldn't normally do. It can cause you to lash out, withdraw, or push away those who love you, even lose who you are. Your emotions become out of balance, they are no longer a well-tuned orchestra, but banging, clashing pots and pans.

Birth trauma can mean at times you are triggered, namely that something will trigger memories that in turn create a strong emotion and then a physical reaction. These can be especially difficult to deal with, as you can feel like you are right back to when the memory happened. Have you ever experienced this with a taste or a smell that has taken you back to a memory perhaps in a favourite restaurant?

When birth is a fearful event your brain makes associations with things that were there at the time and more importantly how it made you feel. Later you are no longer in your birth experience but you may be triggered by anything that reminds you of your birth, which then will also set off the same emotions and physical reaction. For me a huge trigger was my daughter's cry that would transport me back to the hospital ward, the fear would return as would the physical reaction of shaking and a pounding heart.

You can however learn to manage your reaction when you feel an uncomfortable emotion. I can hear you shouting at me saying that you don't believe this because the emotion can feel so overpowering. I can fully understand why because I believed this too! The reactions to my emotions were so strong I couldn't function, my weight plummeted to seven stone because my stomach was so knotted I couldn't eat, and panic attacks would steal my nights till morning broke. Yes, my emotions and the reactions to them definitely kept me hostage and I was paying a heavy toll.

When I became open to my emotions, I learned to embrace them, sit with them and let them be felt knowing why they were here. In time I then began to know and understand my triggers, which in turn allowed me to find ways to prevent them. I quickly realised that for me tiredness was a really big trigger and so I needed to find ways to make sure that I could rest my mind and my body.

As mentioned before my daughter's crying had been a big trigger but by reflecting on why this was the case, namely that I was hurting due to not being with her in those early days, I began to understand that this was something I needed to grieve. It wasn't my fault it was the result of a traumatic birth. This allowed me to add logic to the strong emotions I was feeling. I was able to refocus her crying to realising it was her communicating with me her needs and not a reflection of me as her mother.

Something else that helped me to manage my emotions was having an awareness of what could be called emotional flashbacks. An emotional flashback is when you find you return to the emotional state you experienced during your trauma. It could be fear, panic or abandonment. At these times I would remind myself that this was what was happening. Telling myself that I was in an emotional flashback. That although I felt in danger, I was actually safe. I would name the emotion that I was feeling and why. I would talk soothingly to myself and find ways to ground myself back to the present. I would slow down and find a safe emotional place. Deep breathing would help greatly. Instead of fighting the emotion, I would instead sit with it knowing it was just visiting me for a while like an unwelcome visitor and would eventually leave again.

Unfortunately having emotional flashbacks can cause you to berate yourself and feel like you are failing, or not doing well on your road to healing. Remember that these emotional flashbacks are opportunities to understand that emotion, to see why it is residing with you and to give you the chance to reflect on what you need. Do you need to grieve, or show yourself compassion? Do you need to take time out or ask for help?

It also allows for releasing feelings of panic or fear while you are healing, it supports the processing of difficult memories, and the emotions and physical reactions that they bring back. It means hearing what they are trying to tell you. Emotions that are validated allow for the healing of trauma's wounds.

Embrace your emotions

I have heard it said that some emotions are bad. I don't believe this to be true. I believe that every emotion has a purpose and allows us space to reflect on what it means. It is not the emotion but the actions you take because of that emotion that are good or bad. If you feel angry it may be that it is justified but going and breaking your favourite mug is not. However, anger can be powerful in that it may drive you to get the answers you need about your birth experience, or even to pursue legal action if there was neglect in your care.

So when it comes to emotions whatever they may be, listen to them, what are they whispering to you? Try to understand them and why they are here. Maybe they are telling you that you need to care for yourself more, maybe they are saying that you need to take action. Maybe they are saying today is a day to grieve or to slow down. Whatever your emotions are trying to tell you know that by being open to them they can help you on the road to healing.

It takes bravery and courage to be open to your emotions and it is a hard path to tread, but it pays richly because when you hear and act on what they are trying to tell you, you will find relief from what has been weighing you down. You will find yourself again, knowing that you are no longer held captive by difficult emotions or the physical reactions they evoke. Instead, you are free to continue to walk the road to healing and once again hear the sweet music of your orchestral emotions in balance.

A reflection for you;

Open yourself to your emotions, seek to understand them and in turn, find healing. If you are struggling with an emotion try this exercise.

Name the emotion you are feeling. Reflect on it and try to see where in your body you feel it and how.

- Take a piece of paper and write the emotion in the middle, and write all the things that come to mind that relate to that emotion, such as 'I didn't see my baby', or 'their words were cruel and hurt me'.
- Reflect on what the emotion is trying to tell you about your birth experience. Ask what you know now that you didn't know then. What is the reality of what you faced? What is justified within this emotion and what is instead being viewed through trauma's lens?
- What are some of the physical reactions associated with your emotions? What actions can you take to reduce and support them?
- If you have been triggered try to reflect on what was happening before. Were you overtired, had you done too much, or perhaps you hadn't been showing yourself compassion and self-care? Could you have done anything to prevent it such as resting, asking for help or giving yourself time to work through the difficult emotion?

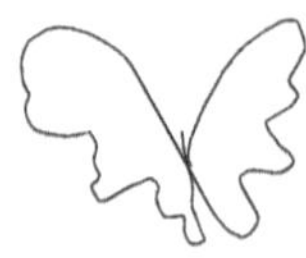

RELAXATION EXERCISE

It is at this point I thought I would mention a relaxation exercise that I use especially when experiencing an emotional flashback.

Find somewhere to sit that is comfortable, where you feel safe and settled. Close your eyes, breathe in deeply and slowly, then exhale and feel the tension leave your body as you do so.

Now imagine yourself as a bright colourful butterfly, as light as a feather, gently fluttering in the breeze. You feel free, nothing can hold you back as you explore the sights and sounds of a beautiful meadow. Feel the warmth of the sun's glow as it warms the earth below you. Take in the scents of the wildflowers, cornflowers, buttercups and daisies as you fly from petal to petal. Notice the blue of the endless sky, clouds wispy like candy floss. In the distance the sound of a nearby stream, draws you closer, bubbling over rocks as you land on a nearby lily pad. In the distance, you can hear the many birds that also share the meadow.

As you take flight again you head to the nearby forest retreating into the cool of tall proud trees. The leaves cause the sunlight to dance and sparkle on the forest floor. You feel the cool of the forest canopy calm you as you come to rest on a fallen log. Linger for a while taking in all the sights and smells of the forest. Allow them to fill your senses and feel the calm they bring. Then slowly let yourself drift up higher and higher up through the trees, into the light, float higher up into the blue of the sky. Then slowly drifting as you return to your chair, to your room. Sit for a moment and notice the calm of your breathing and then slowly open your eyes.

COPING WITH PANIC ATTACKS

"It's hard to fight an enemy that has outposts in your head."
Sally Kempton

The thoughts tumbled and clouded my mind. Fear seized me and I fell that familiar feeling in my stomach. Every part of me was ready to fight an invisible enemy. Pacing steps, drawn breaths, tingling and pain soaring through me. This battle felt too much to bear, it threatened to take me, overwhelm me like the waves of a violent sea. Struggling to keep my head above the water, as the terror tries to pull me under. The voice inside is trying to tell me I'm ok, that I'm safe now, but my body doesn't believe it. I feel lost, out to drift in dark deep waters.

A huge part of my struggle with birth trauma which I found the hardest to deal with was the panic attacks. They are something that plagued me since the birth of my daughter and they were honestly the hardest part of the emotional and physical responses I had to my trauma. They have put me in the hospital many times and have really tested me to the limits of my endurance. I know that many who experience birth trauma also struggle with panic attacks, and they can be truly terrifying. I haven't completely rid myself of panic attacks, I'm not sure I ever will but they are managed, so I thought it may be helpful to share what has helped me.

So what are panic attacks? The media sometimes portrays them as quite light-hearted, and often you will see individuals make flip comments about them, but in reality, they are very serious and can be extremely debilitating to those who suffer from them. They can also accompany emotional flashbacks and cause huge amounts of fear and distress.

For me they start with a strange feeling in my stomach, I often say it feels like icy fingers crawling over me. I shake uncontrollably, have awful nausea and vomiting, my teeth chatter and I get pins and needles all over. I can't keep still, and have an overwhelming urge to walk, or pace often for hours. I'm hot then cold, and find my bladder and bowel cause me more than a little discomfort. I also get intrusive thoughts, this can be about anything, something that is worrying me or has happened recently, they can be thoughts about myself or those I love. I do sometimes hyperventilate too, but not always. My panic attacks can also last for hours, even days as they re-trigger over and over again. I can also experience non-epileptic fits with them which is when I end up with a trip to the hospital. They take a huge toll on me physically and emotionally and it takes me a few days to recover after having one.

What can cause a panic attack? Well, they are a by-product of our natural 'fight or flight response' that nature has given to protect us. For example, if we were threatened by a vicious animal it would cause us to stand and fight or run to try and find safety. I think of it like my natural response has become over-sensitive, as is often the case after suffering trauma. Things that would normally be manageable, instead trigger a meltdown of panic. So what can help to manage panic attacks?

Learn all you can

For me, knowledge has been power. I have done as much research as I can about panic disorder and the fight or flight response. I learnt what the symptoms are, what the hormones involved do to my body and how this affects me. This knowledge armed me with information about what was happening and why, which in turn lessened some of the fear and confusion. Knowing that it was my body and mind reacting to something, helped me to understand why I was responding with panic. Knowing that the symptoms were panic and not that I was desperately ill or dying, also gave me relief and a starting place to try and support myself better.

Know your triggers

For a long time, I didn't understand where the attacks had come from. I used to think they just happened for no reason and this felt like I had no control over them. However, I set about working out why I had a panic attack. I would go over the week or days before and think about what I had been doing or thinking. I soon began to see patterns.

Tiredness was definitely a factor, as was illness in me or others. I have a phobia of vomiting, so feeling nauseous, or others vomiting would set me off. My attacks always happened at night, this was always a mystery to me, so I explored what it was about the night-time that I found hard. I managed to work out that this was related to night times when I was in the hospital after my birth trauma and how this was when I felt my most scared and vulnerable. I have other triggers too and sometimes I get caught out, something on the TV may surprise me and sadly set me off.

Knowing most of my triggers, why they are triggering, and how they affect me, has been a massive turning point. I can't avoid my all my triggers, but I can understand them. This gives back a little control and also helps with the next point, challenging our thoughts.

Challenge your thoughts

Often our own thoughts are what cause our greatest fear. I would often find myself like Alice in Wonderland going down the rabbit hole! One thought would become ten and they would spiral me down into the darkness. Guilt, anger, wondering why me, blaming myself for not being able to cure them, for upsetting others and spoiling things. I would beat myself up in my head and this only served to re-trigger me and make the panic worse.

Challenging these thoughts has been something I have had to really work on and it is still hard. It often feels like a battle in my own head with me as the referee! With practice, it gets easier and it does work, although I find that instead of waiting until I have an attack, challenging negative thoughts is something I must do daily.

Learn to breathe

As I mentioned before I do hyperventilate, but not always. On many occasions well-meaning individuals would say, 'you just need to breathe', usually handing me a paper bag in the process. To be honest this only led to me feeling more nauseous and more triggered. If only it was just that easy!

While for many regulation of breathing is enough to stem their panic, this wasn't enough for me. For me what matters more is being able to calm myself enough to gain back some control, to centre myself and then use the breathing techniques to help create the space to do my other approaches.

It was also important to find a type of breathing exercise that worked. I use a breathing app on my phone that plays a strange sound, that rises and falls to a count of 7 to 4 to 8, with my headphones on it gives me something to focus on, controls my breathing and helps me shut out the cascading thoughts.

I also have a song, 'Blue Ocean Floor', by the lovely Mr. Justin Timberlake. I've no idea why it works but it does, the words have meaning to me, describing how I feel. Whatever the reason, it helps and is part of my coping strategies, helping me to focus and feel calm. I guess the point is that you need to build your own self-care package that supports you to prevent attacks but also to support you when you do have one.

So what else can help during a panic attack? For some grounding techniques help, that bring you back to now, to reality this is especially useful for flashbacks. I have included one in this book for you.

For others distractions can help such as naming all the blue things in the room, counting backwards from 100, or colouring books etc. Others use exercise, meditation and of course medication.

Finding what works for you can take time and perseverance. It can be easy to get discouraged and feel you are not making progress, but you are.

Seek the help of others too. Everyone is different, some wish to battle alone, and others wish someone by their side. For loved ones knowing what to do and how to help can be hard. So at a time when you feel able to, sit down with those you love and tell them what you need to support you. If you support someone who suffers from panic attacks one of the greatest things you can offer is reassurance and love, reminding them that they are ok, that it doesn't change how much you love them and you are there for them can be a source of much-needed comfort.

Panic attacks are very challenging, they can blight your life and at times make life seem impossible. For me, acceptance of them, that I have patches where they return to test me and that sometimes I neglect my self-care has given me the reflection I need to support my well-being. By finding and using what works for me I have been able to reduce them and on the whole live a full life, despite panic being not too far away.

I hope that you can find ways of managing your panic attacks that mean you can enjoy life too. They do not define you, just walk beside you, an unwanted companion that while not a friend, can be managed with a little time, help and hope.

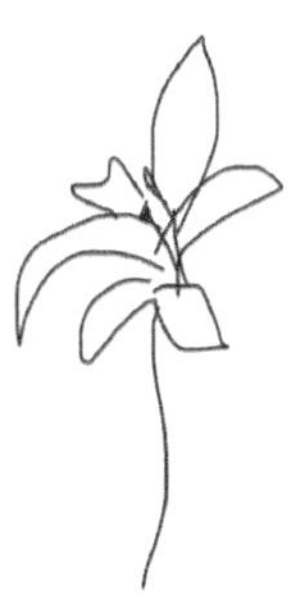

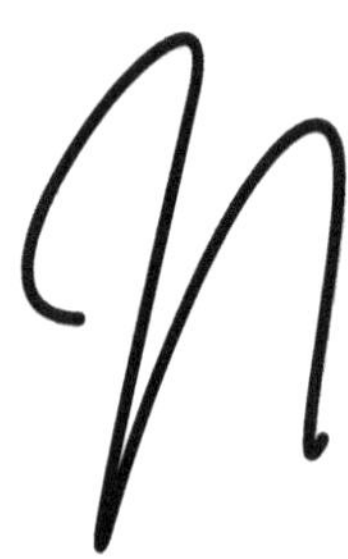

8

N - NOT YOUR FAULT

"And then her heart changed, or at least she understood it, and the winter passed, and the sun shone upon her."
J.R.R. Tolkien

"The hardest thing for me after my birth trauma was the belief that it was my fault, that somehow I could have prevented it and this haunted me."
Louise

One of the hardest aspects regarding birth trauma is accepting that what happened was not your fault. However to heal beyond birth trauma and to keep going on the road to healing, understanding and accepting that birth trauma is not your fault is a huge stone that you need to climb over.

Oh, but I can hear you say, 'If only I had done this, or that, or if I had stood up for myself or believed in myself more then maybe it would have been different, or never have happened at all'.

I believed for a long time that my traumatic birth experience was all my fault. I lost myself in the belief that I was somehow to blame and it cocooned me in a darkness that was hard to break out of. When you believe that trauma is your fault it breaks your belief in yourself. It causes shame, guilt and endless what-ifs. It also causes you to second guess all your choices including ones you made in the past but also the ones you are making now and for the future. I found this to be true. In my darkest times, I would replay my pregnancy and birth over and over again, looking for the smallest thing that I should have said or done differently. I sought to find ways to play a different version of the events that had befallen me only to cause myself more pain in the process.

My journey of pregnancy with my first daughter wasn't easy. To be honest I wasn't sure she would ever arrive, after a year of trying to get pregnant I began to wonder if it just wasn't going to happen for me. I remember sitting outside the doctor's office waiting to be seen, wondering what he would say and what options lay ahead. I sat, waiting, glossy magazines lay on the table with celebrity lives for all to see, my mouth dry and my hands shaking. When I finally saw the doctor, he made it seem like this was all very routine and gave me a small tablet that he guaranteed would give me what I was hoping for, a baby.

So sure enough about two months later the day my period was due and unable to wait a day longer, I took the test and there it was, those two tiny blue lines indicating it had worked and that yes, I was pregnant. That meant a baby, a real baby was growing right now, this minute, inside me. I pretty much carried on as normal the next few weeks, feeling happy at the little secret my belly was hiding.

It was a Saturday night and I had been to a party, I had sat quietly all evening resisting the pull of others to dance and when we finally got home I felt especially exhausted. I woke in the middle of the night and felt strange, I couldn't tell you how, but I just knew something was wrong. I turned over in bed, it felt wet, and when I turned on the light and I looked beneath the covers, they were scarlet red with blood. I heard the call to the ambulance, saw the faces of the paramedics above me, and the lights on the roof of the ambulance as it winged its way to the hospital but I was consumed with the voice in my head that kept saying my baby was gone.

Night time in the hospital was strange, the ward was quiet, in an eerie way, finally the porters came for me at 9.00 am with a big wheelchair and wheeled me across the bumpy carpark to the antenatal clinic for a scan. I sat in the wheelchair, shaking with cold and fear, listening to the porters discuss the news and football. What had I done wrong to be sitting here, crying silent tears alone, waiting? As I was wheeled into the room, it wasn't how I'd expected my first scan to be. It was supposed to be an exciting time, to see my baby, trace its outline, laugh and cry at its tiny form, and walk away with my picture to show friends and family, instead, I was sat waiting to see if all was lost. The jelly was cold, the scanner rolled over my belly, and I held my breath, I didn't look at the screen but fixed my gaze on a poster talking about folic acid. Only the clicks of the machine broke the silence. It seemed like an eternity before a voice broke the silence, making me jump and telling me to look at the screen where I saw in black and white a tiny heart beating away.

The doctor came later that day to tell me that I had been carrying twins and that I had lost one of my babies. I went home that day, still bleeding but thankful of the tiny heart beating inside me. Over the next few weeks, however, anxiety was very much taking hold and I obsessed about why my pregnancy was threatened. Was it my fault, should I not have attended the party, was it the medication I took to help me get pregnant? I had already lost one baby and I desperately sought to keep the tiny life inside me safe.

I did bleed again in my pregnancy, not as bad as the first time, but still enough to raise concern, yet the scans showed a healthy, growing baby. However, at 34 weeks pre-eclampsia threatened to take both our lives and so my baby was delivered in the most traumatic of circumstances. My aftercare also added much to the trauma I already felt and again I would torture myself about had this all been my fault. I felt such pain that my body had not been able to protect my baby. For me, pregnancy was a time of loss, and my birth a time of trauma.

Over my journey of healing, I have come to see that my pregnancy and birth experiences were not my fault, but it took a long time to accept this. I use to question everything, did I do anything that caused the loss of my daughter's twin? What about the bleeding and then the pre-eclampsia and my baby being born early? Did I do anything that caused my placenta to get stuck or the haemorrhage that nearly took me? Why did I have such awful cruel care, was I hard to care for, what did I do to cause them to treat me that way? Was it my fault that we lost all those first moments, that my baby lay in neonatal?

After years of torturing myself, I have over time been able to find peace that it wasn't my fault and that sometimes circumstances befall us that we can do nothing about.

Sometimes pregnancy is a time of loss and sadly something many parents experience. We still don't know why so many women miscarry but the pain is real and devastating to all. It wasn't the party I attended, or that I hadn't rested or anything else my mind tried to convince me of, but for reasons I will never know I lost the twin to my daughter. It wasn't my fault I had pre-eclampsia and had to save our lives by delivering my baby into the world when she wasn't yet ready. It wasn't my fault that her birth was an emergency, that required life-saving surgery, or that the care I received after giving birth left me hurt and broken, an empty shell. It wasn't my fault that our maternity journey had been hard and as a result, left me traumatised.

How can you come to understand that your birth trauma wasn't your fault? By taking time to see that you did the best you could, at a time when you were feeling scared and vulnerable and with the best knowledge you had available to you, in likely very difficult circumstances. That when you look back you do so with hindsight as your friend, with knowledge that you have now, but didn't have then. It is true also that with all the will in the world so much of life is out of our control and this is true of birth too. Birth is complex and so are you. There are so many variables and so many things that can in change pregnancy and birth.

I want you to know that it wasn't your fault if you suffered poor care. You weren't a difficult patient or demanding. The care given is the responsibility of the caregiver. Women in birth are vulnerable and need compassion and kindness. You deserved to have care that protected you and made you feel safe. Care that reflected compassion and empathy. Care that respected you and your needs and afforded you dignity. The fault instead lies with those that didn't offer you comfort, pain relief, or simply a hand to hold.

It wasn't your fault that you weren't listened to when you tried to say what you needed or when you spoke up about what you didn't want to happen or that you were feeling scared and in pain. That you weren't offered choices that could have helped you feel more in control of your birth or that your choices were not respected but instead discarded as of no importance. Neither was it your fault that when you tried to speak up and advocate for yourself this was ignored and instead you were left feeling abandoned and silenced.

It wasn't your fault that individuals chose to use language to you that caused you pain, stabbing like a knife, wounding your soul and hurting the very fabric of who you are. That disregarded your identity or wishes. That lacked empathy or understanding. That disregarded your feelings, your beliefs or your culture. That made you feel a burden or alone. It wasn't your fault that you were neglected physically and/or emotionally. That no one saw you, no one heard you, no one came when you needed them. That your concerns were dismissed or your cries for help ignored.

It was not your fault that you lost a much-wanted birth experience. That all your hopes and dreams feel broken into pieces. That grief feels heavy and the loss too much to bear. That the birth of your baby was traumatic and has left you struggling to make sense of everything. That it wasn't what you had hoped and dreamed of, that the things that meant so much were stolen away.

Whatever the reason you feel that birth trauma was your fault, hear me when I tell you that this is just not true. Trauma lies to us. Do not let the voice of trauma whisper to you and cause you to believe that it was your fault.

You endured a traumatic event, that happened beyond your control, and you did all you could to survive. You did everything you could to protect your baby, to protect yourself. You could not control how others behaved, or how they treated you. You could not control the fact that sometimes birth becomes complex, or an emergency or not how you had hoped.

It is true also that sometimes pregnancy and birth mean the making of choices that are hard and can cause you pain and distress. Maybe it is if a pregnancy should continue, or that medical help may be needed to keep you both safe. There can be times when the choices you made were the right choice for you and your family but still caused you pain and trauma. This again was not your fault. Birth is a place of vulnerability and however right the choice may be it can still affect you. You didn't feel trauma because you made a choice, but because that choice was profound and you are a human being, with feelings that can feel the rawness that sometimes life brings to your door. No birth trauma was not your fault.

Can preparation for birth prevent birth trauma?

There has been talk in the birthing world about how if we prepare women for birth, we prevent birth trauma. Many women I have supported over the years have voiced to me that they have felt their birth has been traumatic because they didn't prepare enough for it and so the trauma they feel was their fault.

When I trained as a Birth Buddy I learnt how important it is that women are helped to understand the physiology of birth, how they can work with their bodies to birth their baby and that they are given support to have a positive birth experience. However, does this and other techniques such as hypo-birthing prevent women from experiencing birth trauma?

Without a doubt preparation for birth matters. It supports you to make informed choices, it helps to build trust with those who will care for you, and it should also help prepare you for if things don't go to plan, or situations arise that mean a change to your birth plan or your wishes.

Preparation for birth may take many forms, it may be antenatal education, birthing classes, self-education or support in the form of a doula or other birth worker. Preparation should be individual and tailored to a family's needs and circumstances. For instance, preparation will be different for a woman who plans a water birth to a woman planning a caesarean.

It is important that choice is supported in any antenatal preparation, and that parents understand the birth they have planned and how this may impact them after. It should also address the emotional side of birth not just the medical and how when birth is difficult the impact can be profound. That the transition to parenthood is hard too. Does this though prevent a woman from feeling traumatised from a difficult birth experience?

Trauma felt after birth is very individual because birth is individual to each woman. Every experience you go through in life will affect you differently and you may react to it differently than someone else who has had a similar experience. This is because we all have different previous life experiences, cultures, beliefs and current life circumstances. What matters is how each woman feels about 'her' birth experience. So what about the claim that preparing for birth prevents birth trauma?

The question is can you truly prepare for something that you haven't yet experienced or know how it will affect you? Of course not. You can do everything possible to make sure you do what you can to be ready to face any situation in life, but the reality is that life including birth is unpredictable. With all the best preparation in the world when thrown into an emergency, when confronted by a situation that places you or your loved ones in danger, the effect on you and those around you can be profound and life-changing. This applies to birth too.

Also by saying that women can prepare to prevent being traumatised, we put the onus on women, we say that they have the responsibility to prevent being traumatised, yet is this really something that she can control? A woman no matter how prepared she may be for birth cannot prepare for when trauma is caused by poor care, cruel language, or medical neglect. This is out of her control.

Preparing a woman for her birth doesn't mean that she should be accepting of care that is damaging to her or her baby. It doesn't mean that she should somehow be resilient against care that is neglectful. Rather care given should be protective of women and their partners so that even in the most difficult of situations choice and support for them is possible.

It is true too that nothing can prepare families for the physical damage that may result from a difficult birth to a woman or her baby, the time spent in a neonatal unit or sadly if a woman loses her baby.

Also by claiming that preparation before birth prevents birth trauma, we can then induce guilt and silence those that do feel traumatised. Blame is a huge part of feeling traumatised as we have already seen. If a woman feels she didn't do enough to prepare, if she feels that something she did or didn't do could have prevented her birth trauma then we place blame at her feet. This only perpetuates the cycle of guilt and the belief that a woman somehow caused her trauma, that it is her fault or that she should have been stronger, more resilient, or more accepting of the trauma she has been through. Women are not to blame and never should this be suggested.

Of the many women I have supported who have suffered from birth trauma it is very clear that they are often the strongest, most resilient, brave and courageous people I have ever met. Despite their experiences, the pain they endure physically as well as emotionally, and despite having little in the way of support or understanding, they fight every day to care for their families, go to work and cope with the impact birth trauma has thrust upon them.

When we think of the many things that can cause trauma such as natural disasters, terrorist attacks, and abuse in its many forms would we ever suggest that individuals can prepare to prevent feeling traumatised or that they should have coped with it better? Of course not, so why do we suggest this about birth?

At this point, it is also important to mention that there are some women who are more predisposed to suffer trauma from birth due to previous trauma such as rape or child abuse. For women who may have a history of trauma from whatever source, care that is trauma-informed is vital. Care that is respectful and maintains dignity, that provides emotional support during pregnancy and birth is what will help reduce the possibility of re-traumatising or adding to previous trauma. Many who have endured abuse will carry the narrative that the awful events that have happened to them in their life are in some way their fault. While it may be true that previous trauma may make some more likely to be triggered during pregnancy and birth, the onus is upon those giving care to reduce the possibility of this leading to birth trauma. Never should it be the case that women believe their birth to be another traumatic event for which they are to blame or that they in some way should have prevented it.

It's true also that many women voice that they feel they did prepare for their birth even attended classes to support the way they wished to birth and have then felt disappointed that this wasn't their experience. This again is where caution is needed in saying we can prepare women for birth.

When the preparation is focused on one way of birth, doesn't reflect the honest complexity of birth or tells women that their birth will go well if they just trust and believe in their bodies, then we are leaving the way open to cause harm. When birth is then traumatic women will look to blame themselves, thinking they didn't believe in themselves enough or trust in their bodies enough or worse that they somehow failed, or their bodies failed or they failed their babies.. No woman fails when she births her baby and never should she feel that her difficult experience is her fault.

So what can help to reduce birth trauma for women and their partners? We will discuss this in more detail in a later chapter. While helping parents to be prepared for birth is important, birth is complex and individual and preparation isn't how we fully prevent birth from being traumatic.

What I do know is that I've had so many families share with me that it was the support and good care they received that helped to prevent even in the most difficult of situations, trauma from taking hold. The care given to women when kind, compassionate and respectful while protecting dignity helps reduce trauma. It should be individual and take into account the individual's history and personal circumstances. It should allow for and respect choice, even in emergency situations, so that women can feel that they are still in control and part of their care plan. Emotional support should be given just as much emphasis as physical care. It should include communication that is respectful and clear and allows women to make informed choices about their care. Also, specialist support should be given to families that suffer maternal or infant damage, have a baby in a neonatal unit or lose their babies.

Birth trauma may never be completely prevented but there is plenty that can be done to reduce it or support those affected when it does happen.

Preparation has its place in helping families in birth, but when trauma happens it is not because this preparation didn't happen or didn't work. Rather that traumatic events happen even in birth, just as they happen in life. Rather than lay the blame on women for birth being traumatic or suggest that they could have prevented it, may we instead hear what they have to say. With the acceptance that birth can be unpredictable, we can lessen the impact of birth trauma on families by helping them feel safe, supported, and cared for.

Say it with me. It wasn't your fault!

Is the voice of birth trauma whispering to you? Is it causing you to doubt yourself and believe that it was somehow your fault? If it is it's time to now silence it. Birth trauma was not your fault. When the voice of trauma tries to make you believe otherwise know that it is lying to you. Take this truth down into your heart and believe it with every fibre in your being.

The truth is you did the best you could at a time when it felt like your world was falling apart when you were vulnerable and scared. You are more brave than you could possibly know and I see you. Don't let this hold you back as you walk your road to healing, instead, take my hand, see the stone before you and climb right over it, as you do so lift your eyes and see your destination to healing ahead.

A reflection for you;

- Take a piece of paper and on the right-hand side write down the things that birth trauma is whispering to you to make you believe it was somehow your fault. Then allow yourself to feel compassion for the You that was present at your birth almost like you are a third person in the room. What would you like the You back then to know?
- Now write down a reply to the things that birth trauma is whispering to you. (Here is an example; 'I shouldn't have let myself be treated so unkindly' to 'I had no control over how others treated me.')
- *The Birth Bill of Rights.* Right a list of what your 'rights' were for how you should have been treated at your birth.

Here are a few examples;

1. I had the right to be treated with respect.
2. I had the right to be informed about what was happening to me.
3. I had the right to say NO.
4. I had the right to care that was compassionate.

Really ponder on these and allow them to show you that your birth trauma was not your fault. That you deserved a birth that kept you both physically and emotionally safe.

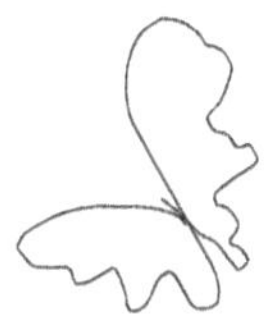

POEM
I DIDN'T SUFFER BIRTH TRAUMA
BECAUSE…

I didn't suffer birth trauma because I was…
Uninformed
Or lacking in knowledge or information

Because I didn't have…
Soft music
Candles
Or dim lights

Or because I didn't…
Pray
Meditate
Use affirmations
Be active
Read enough
Plan enough

Or because I needed…
Medical interventions
Pain relief
Or to be in the hospital

Or because I was weak, or unprepared.

I suffered birth trauma because…
I was treated like a nuisance
Not communicated with
Berated for my choices
Ignored
Belittled
Dismissed
Bombarded with cruel words

Because I was…
Slapped
Held down
Lied to
Sneered at
Laughed at
Neglected
Abandoned
Called names

I lost things that were precious to me.

I suffered birth trauma because I was not treated with kindness and dignity, instead hurt physically and emotionally.

I suffered birth trauma because I was nearly taken from this world, from my family and my baby was nearly taken too.

There was nothing to keep me safe emotionally, no one to care for me and ease me when death sought me to embrace.

Birth trauma was not my fault.

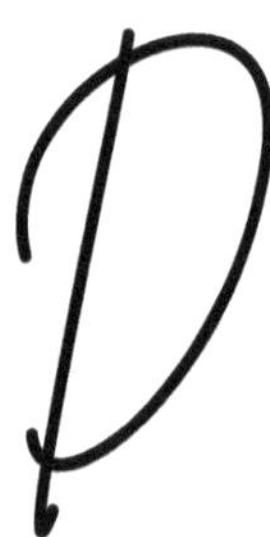

9

D -DO NOT GIVE UP

"Although the world is full of suffering, it is full also of the overcoming of it."
Helen Keller

"Trying to recover from birth trauma was hard, there were days when I thought I just can't do this."
Nazim

DO NOT GIVE UP

Even when the days are dark.
Do not give up.
When you feel that you can't carry on.
Do not give up.
When the feelings are overwhelming.
Do not give up.
When you doubt you can heal beyond birth trauma.
Do not give up.

This is the smallest chapter in the book but so very important. I guarantee you there will be days on your journey to healing when you will feel you just can't carry on. Instead, you will sit down, weary, not knowing where the strength will come from to pick yourself up again. The road may feel blocked, or like walking on sharp rocks. Maybe the road ahead feels so long and hard that you can't see any light on the horizon. Maybe a thick fog blocks you're sight and you feel like you are wandering around lost. I had many of these days on my road to healing. Days when I longed for peace to return, when I longed to be released from birth traumas grip. To find me again and to enjoy my family, my life.

Birth trauma made me feel like my life had been stolen. Precious moments measured in minutes, hours, days and weeks lost to a thief that freely wandered into my life with no regard for the things I held dear. My thief had no face, just darkness that crept in and overshadowed me.

I would think about the days I had lost, of special moments that could have been, but instead, my thief had taken them, leaving hollow sadness where memories should have been. My thief made my fragile heart pound till it felt like it would stop for all eternity. My stomach my thief made toss, turn and crash like the powerful waves of the sea. In my head thoughts that I was unlovable, a burden to those I loved, my thief conjured like a magician. Weakness became my companion and tiredness my confidant. All around me became a blur. A sea of faces laughing, smiling at life as it should be. I felt like I was gasping for air, for my thief had stolen my breath, its hands at my throat. Burning tears stung my eyes while I looked for hope, for peace. Smiling photographs hid pain and sorrow but in my eyes only the thief's reflection. A painted face tried to hide the stricken pallor that testified to the constant battle I waged. I longed to banish it, my thief, to lock all the doors to my mind and heart throwing away the key. But it always found a way to evade my protection and spread its darkness again. Many times it made me believe that everyone was better off without me. I felt lost, my road ahead covered in a thick suffocating fog.

Like me, there are so many who also have their own thief, created by their birth experience. I see the pain etched on their faces daily. Birth trauma makes them believe that life has been stolen, light has been taken over by darkness and hope no longer exists. Maybe this is how you are feeling too right now as you hold this book in your trembling hands.

If you are reading this and feeling that you have lost your way, please hold on. Don't give up. I know it's hard I've been there hanging on by my fingertips. I want you to know that you can do this and that you can find your way again.

If you find that things are overwhelming take some time to see what can help you. You may need to rest a while on your journey and this is ok. Resting both physically and mentally has huge benefits to healing and can allow space to reflect on your next steps. Resting the mind allows for healing and can be needed especially if triggers have been abundant.

Maybe you need to ask for help, be it from friends and family or from professionals who can provide the right therapy and support be it practically and/or emotionally. This can be hard especially if you have been traveling your road and felt like you have been making good progress. Remember that help is part of healing and reaching out to those who can provide it is needed as you continue to walk your road.

Maybe you need to stop and search again to see what it is you need at this point on your journey to help you see past the fog that is clouding your view. Also, stop and look behind you at how far you have already travelled and all that you have overcome so it can strengthen you to carry on.

You may be torn and twisted as you try to navigate your road, sometimes it takes winding detours that seek to lead you away from your destination. While you may feel like giving up and the road may feel never-ending, those detours can sometimes be good, as they lead us to places that bring healing from unexpected sources.

Allow yourself time, to take stock and let this instead be a time for reflection. Try to use this space to see how to can find your way again and where you can go next. Never feel like you are not making progress because you are.

While your thief has taken so much from you, it is possible to recover and heal beyond birth trauma. I know this because I've walked the same road, I've stumbled, fallen, been lost in the fog and at times crawled my road on my hands and knees. I promise you it is a road you can successfully walk to your destination of healing. Progress is sometimes beyond your vision, you can't see it because you are in the thick of it like walking through a patch of dense forest. Progress though is always there in some way, even if it is just understanding the impact that this is having on you. Progress may appear to you to be invisible but it is there, just keep going.

What can help you not to give up on your road to healing and recovery?

I've spoken a lot about the right support and again I must say how vital it is and how it was a very important part of my recovery. Seek help and lean on those who can encourage you while you're healing. You may find this in friends, family, support groups, social media or even with strangers. More importantly, let yourself be helped. I know you want to do this on your own, I know you may feel like you shouldn't need anyone's help but this will only cause your healing to take longer. Your trust in others may have been broken because trauma damages your connections to others and your sense of safety. Know that you are surrounded by those who love you, they want to be there to offer whatever they can to help you. Slowly build your trust again with those who reach out to you, who want to support you and let them be a help, even guide on your road.

Don't forget to ask for practical help. Even help with the small things and the hectic parts of life can make a huge difference. Trying to carry on without the needed support can lead you to exhaustion and make you feel like giving up. Practical help can take many forms and you will know what is helpful to you and your circumstances. No one can walk this road without the help of others.

Make a self-care tool bag to help you stay strong and keep you going even on bad days. I do struggle with the term 'self-care' because it can conjure up images of things you may think are just not realistic. Personally, I like to think of it as all the things that help you keep going on your road. It can be anything that brings you calm and helps you to feel restored again. It can be a walk, a favourite boxset, a talk with a friend or letting out your creative side. It can be a cuddle with your cat or a funny video on TV. When I was unwell with birth trauma self-care was something that felt too overwhelming. As I began to recover I remember the day that I felt able to just paint my nails, it was such a small thing, something I had taken for granted before but something that I hadn't been able to do because trauma had been so impacting my mind. Those pretty sparkly nails were a sign to me, a small sign of hope that I was beginning to heal, to find myself again, a reminder that I mattered and part of that, was caring for myself physically too.

When you feel like you want to give up take a look behind you and see how far you have come, use this to spur you on to keep going, to lift and support you as you heal. Small steps are still steps and they should never be dismissed. Instead let them encourage you to look to the future, to take even more small steps with hope, realising that your birth trauma doesn't have to define you, or control you. Remind yourself that while you have been hurt by birth trauma, and even though you may feel it has stolen so much from you, you have also made so much progress on your road and you can keep taking more steps to healing.

As the quote for this chapter expressed there is much suffering especially when it comes to birth trauma, yet I have with my own eyes seen and have experienced the ability to overcome it.

Whenever I talk to families who are suffering after birth trauma I wish that I held a magic wand that I could use to wipe away all their pain and heartache and carry them to the end of their road to healing. I wish also that I could use it to make birth trauma a thing of the past. Sadly this just isn't a reality. However, what moved and drove me to write this book was that I wanted to give hope. Hope that no matter what you have endured, how deeply you have been affected, no matter how much you have lost, or how heavy your sadness, you can find healing. That while you may still have bad days this doesn't mean you are not on your way to recovery.

Yes, just like you I have been at the point of wanting to give up. Yet I'm here, speaking to you through the pages of this book. As I look back I'm so grateful that I held on, sometimes with my fingertips. I have been able to build new memories and experiences with my daughters, I have watched them grow, felt their love and found my worth as their mum. I have built friendships with others that I would never have met had it not been for my journey. Friendships that have given me strength, and solace and taught me so much. I have also been able to offer help and support to others who like me have been touched by birth trauma.

I didn't ask for this journey and neither have you, yet we are here and together we can help each other. I wish I could reach out of this book and hug you, and sit alongside you to let you know it will be ok. Instead, I hope the words on this page can speak to your heart and gently encourage you to carry on. You are so very precious, never let birth trauma make you believe otherwise.

So don't give up! You can heal beyond birth trauma. Yes it will be hard, and yes it will mean finding strength that you never thought possible but I know that what you need to heal is right there within you.

You have changed, indeed your life may have changed, but this is not the end of your story. You are starting to write a new chapter, that will be different, new, and challenging but definitely brighter. You are still you, and just as amazing as before birth trauma touched you, in fact, more so, because despite everything you are walking your road to healing, overcoming all the obstacles it has thrown at you and I know you will come out the other side.

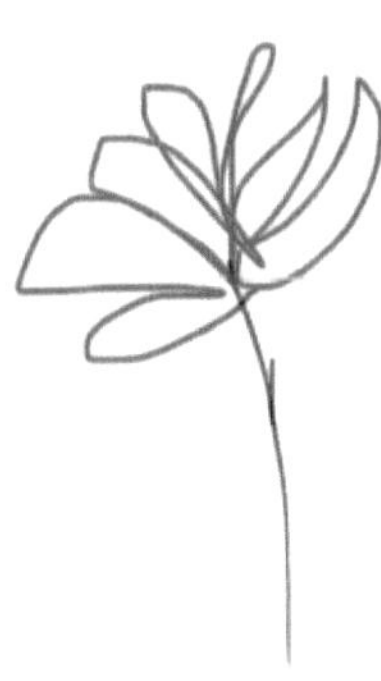

A reflection for you;

When we go through something traumatic it is like we have been shattered into many pieces and we may feel broken. Healing means gathering all those pieces of you back together again to help you feel whole.

- Take a piece of paper and draw you in the middle or write your name. Then taking brightly coloured pens write all around it who you are. There will be the roles you fill such as mother or daughter. There will be the talents you possess, maybe you are creative or musical, the gifts you hold such as a sense of justice, and the qualities you show, such as love and kindness. Ask friends and family too, what they admire and love about you and add them to your picture. These are the pieces of you.

- Then imagine all these brightly coloured pieces coming back together. Let the pieces form a beautiful, colourful kaleidoscope. See how these pieces are what defines you, not what happened to you. You are not your trauma, you are the beautiful merging of all these pieces, these are what makes you, YOU. Put your picture up somewhere so that you can see it every day. Let it give you hope, strength and determination to keep going on your journey beyond birth trauma.

10

HOPE, RECOVERY AND GROWTH

"Under the cloak of winter, a snowdrop lies buried deep. It is a promise of tomorrow, in life and growth, from the darkest of places, to find the warmth of spring again."

"I never believed that recovery was possible, put in time not only did I see recovery was possible but so much more."
Sarah

Some days the darkness was overwhelming. I felt like a dark cloud was my daily companion and no matter what I did, it would not leave my side. I looked at everyone else and longed to be like them. To me, they seemed bathed in sunshine, a glorious light that was happiness and joy. I felt alone, an outcast who sought the warmth of others while at the same time believing all I could offer them was sadness. The face I painted on each day, and the clean, perfectly ironed clothes, only sought to hold my lie more captive. I was suffering, hope felt lost.

Finding hope

The days, weeks and months after birth that are difficult or traumatic can be cast in darkness. Each day can be a battle, thoughts in your head seeking to drive you to the brink of despair. I used to liken it to being in a bubble, everything was muffled by my experience, tainted and impaired. The air around me felt suffocating, I longed to escape the thoughts in my head and the visions that visited me. Numbness often accompanied the darkness, a way to cope, to keep going. This meant moments lost, and memories stolen, as merely existing became the aim. Light felt snuffed out and along with it hope.

Yet as I began to walk my road to recovery I soon saw that even in the darkest of times there were moments of light to be found. These moments of light could be fleeting, only seconds, small prisms that poked a hole through the clouds but with them they brought hope.

What are moments of light? These moments are individual to you. They are anything that lifts the clouds no matter how momentary. It can be a smile or a kind word from a loved one or a stranger. They can be your little ones' embrace or a funny little thing they do that touches your heart. It can be a chat with a friend, or a cup of tea and a moment of peace. It can be a crisp autumn morning, the warm sun of a summer's day or standing in awe as a sunset stains the sky. It may be a small achievement as you navigate your road. Or reconnection with your partner. It may be that your moment of light is gaining back those pieces of you that you feel have been lost.

It isn't what your moment is, it is seeing them that counts. You may need to search, in fact, search deeply for your moments of light. On days that are overwhelmingly dark, you may think that there are no moments, no light to break through. Finding your moments of light is a deeply personal journey and they are important as these moments are what give hope. Like prisms, they reflect light that can be seen from many angles and in many colours. The more we see them the more they break through the clouds of birth trauma.

Living with the aftermath of what you have been through can convince your mind to only look for danger, for things that may be harmful to you both physically and emotionally. Before long this can become your 'norm', till all that is good, all that you are achieving each day is missed, lost as if obscured from view by a deep cloud. Soon you become good at always missing that you are a good parent, who is doing everything you can to care for and love your family.

My hardest times as I mentioned before have always been at night. After busy days that served in some way to distract me, when calm and quiet descended at night my mind would turn on itself. All my worries and anxieties would plague me and cause me to dwell on how I believed I failing at everything. While darkness was outside, it was nothing compared to the darkness that was filling my mind. I began to dread night falling, and panic would often ensue.

I decided that I had to somehow change the narrative. So each night I would try to let my mind find one thing that I could take from the day no matter how small, that was a moment of light. I would focus on it and let it fill my thoughts, that moment being the thing I saw when I closed my eyes. Sometimes it was just surviving, just getting dressed or managing a meal. To me, they were small victories, small moments that gave me hope, that broke the seemingly impenetrable blackness. Something then began to happen. It became easier to find my moments of light. Instead of the belief that all that surrounded me was only darkness, I saw there was in fact light too. The more that I believed this, the more I sought out these moments and the more they shone brightly.

As the light found me and reflected the bright colours of hope, I also found belief in myself. I was doing better than I had given myself credit for and stronger than I dared to believe. While my birth experience had tainted my world I was starting to see beyond it.

I started to see that I was healing, I was taking small steps to my destination. Moments of light led to the belief that recovery was possible and so stronger hope, which in turn led to determination to keep going on my road.

There are many ways to seek and grasp your moments of light. Memory jars are great to collect moments over a week, month or year. Writing down these moments, putting them into a jar and then reading them back to yourself can be powerful and encouraging. Another way is to have a journal, there are many available to choose from but the ones I really like encourage you to write something each day that has inspired, comforted, strengthened or been positive for you.

Photography to me has been a way to capture my moments of light. Nature has so much to offer us and dwelling on the beauty it displays has been so healing to me. Capturing moments, a video of your little one laughing or your pet doing something funny can be replayed to give light on days when darkness seems to prevail. Finding your moments of light is a deeply personal journey. So seek them out you may surprised by what you find.

It can be emotionally strengthening to see that your darkest days do have moments of light. It will be hard at first to find them but do not give up. These moments are gifts that give hope and support healing. So grasp the moments, hold on to them with all your might, and let them support you on your road to healing.

Growth after birth Trauma

The dark days of winter seem endless. Before the vernal equinox, while cold winds cut deep and winters bite still holds tight its grip, the assurance of spring and the return of light and brighter days are promised by the welcome sight of barren ground covered in a carpet of small white flowers – Snowdrops. These tiny flowers are givers of hope. The first to bloom forth from the ravages of winter. A tiny bulb buried deep in dark, cold, soil, pushes forth from land that has lain dormant under frost and snow, to reveal a delicate flower. Then these beautiful snowdrops amass together, creating such a beautiful spectacle that people travel from afar to look upon their beauty.

Snowdrops teach us much about healing and strength, hope and endurance, as well as the power of support. This relates so much to healing from birth trauma.

The time after birth trauma can be dark and hostile. As we have already seen you can feel alone, abandoned and isolated. You can feel buried by emotions and feelings you may not understand, often overwhelmed at the weight this places on you. Like a tiny snowdrop, you can feel like you are buried deep in birth trauma's soil. Light is nowhere to be found and the coldness of the isolation felt can leave you feeling frozen, unable to see a way out or to feel any hope. Even managing daily life itself may feel impossible. Yet we can learn so much from snowdrops.

Tiny snowdrops find the strength to search for the smallest amount of warmth and light that grace cold, dark, winter days. They know that with strength and perseverance, they can push through the dark ground and bloom forth for all to see. So too, despite the depths of birth trauma's grip you can find the strength to push through, to find light and hope again, and grow beyond it.

This may feel impossible to you right now. You may feel fragile, broken and engulfed in the sadness of what you have experienced. Yet, have you ever picked a snowdrop, held it in your hands and felt its petals? They are the most gentle of flowers, soft and delicate and yet are able to withstand the hardest of winters and bloom when spring is only just beginning. You are like a snowdrop. While feeling fragile and vulnerable you also hold within you incredible strength, determination and ability for growth. You have already shown this to be true every day as you continue to try and deal with everything birth trauma has thrown at you.

Recovery may at this point seem hard to you and growth after trauma impossible. I want you to know that it is possible. It will take courage to believe that finding any light and life again will be something you can reach. Little by little, you will push forward through the darkness, each day you will reach a little further forward. This takes time and hard work, after all the weight of birth trauma is heavy.

As snowdrops seek to break free from the cold soil, they begin to feel any warmth the winter sun casts on the ground, this encourages them more, and soon they also feel the light spring rains that soften them and the ground providing nourishment. As you endeavour to recover and grow again after birth trauma, encouragement will come in many forms. It will come from those small achievements or your moments of light, from the kind words of loved ones that ease painful thoughts, and the building back of trust and connection with others that birth trauma sought to pull down. These are warming to you like a spring sun, giving you strength as you realise that your experience doesn't define or control you.

So too the rain of self-care and support in whatever way that may be found can nourish you and help you to continue to push forward. This is growth, it is new life, a change from what was before. It is the acceptance that new life means change, and while you may have been changed by your experience, there is still so much of life to embrace.

As the snowdrop reaches the surface and breaks forth, it still has battles to face. Fine and fragile, the land is still cold, yet the snowdrop is determined. It knows that soon spring with its warmth and new life will return and it is part of the journey that heralds it. It knows its worth, and what it brings to nature and the world. The snowdrop knows too that it is not alone, for all around are many snowdrops who also are pushing forth to find the sun. These amass together to give more strength to each other, providing shelter and protection as they battle the passing of winter.

You also will continue to fight many battles as you try to heal and grow after birth trauma but do not doubt your ability to do so. Look at what you have overcome so far, you are a beautiful complexity of vulnerability and strength just like a snowdrop. Also, know your worth. What you mean to those who love you, what gifts and abilities you bring to the world, what others see in you as you continue to wage your battle against birth trauma.

Use also the strength that comes from others who like you are seeking to break free from the weight of birth trauma's grip. Just as snowdrops stand together to battle the biting winds and cold frosts, find those that will stand by your side, giving you shelter and protection against trauma's winter. It will surprise you to know how many others like you struggle with how their baby's birth has impacted them. There is solace and companionship to be found. As we all stand together, it leaves everyone in awe and creates the most beautiful spectacle that will make others stop and look in wonder. It also gives hope to the many others affected, helping them to break free, knowing that hope is powerful and healing possible as they too bloom just like a snowdrop.

It is said in myth that snowdrops are a powerful herb antidote to poison. While snowdrops may eventually fade to give way to the emergence of spring, their power can remain. The power they carry can fight off the poison that seeks to take life. Your hope, strength and determination can just like the snowdrop, fight birth trauma's poison. Instead of halting life, it gives life, new life that while may have changed, has so much to offer.

For me, growth came slowly, but it did come. I learnt ways to cope and understand my experience as I've shared in the pages of this book. I went on to find ways to channel all that I had been through so I could heal, grow and eventually help others. I believe that we go through things in life that change us, that rock us to our very core but even the bad can be used for good. I never wished for this journey, but it was one that I had to travel. My wish is that in some small way, my sharing my journey will help you too.

So when you can go take a look, go gaze upon the carpets of snowdrops that cover the earth in spring. Let their beauty fill you with strength and hope. Just like a snowdrop, you can break free of birth trauma's grip. You can grow and show your beauty while giving hope to others as you do so. Just as the snowdrop assures us of spring's return, or life starting a new one, so too you can find life and healing beyond birth trauma.

Happy Birthday, Little One!

All around are bright coloured balloons, the cake waiting for candles to be lit and wishes to be made. Gifts wrapped in shiny paper call out to be opened. Deep inside turmoil churns away. Today is supposed to be happy, a celebration, but instead, there is pain, sorrow and sadness. This isn't supposed to be how you feel today, the birthday of your dear little one.

One thing I get asked about a lot is the birthday of your baby which can be a challenge when seeking to heal from birth trauma. The conflict of emotions felt can be deeply troubling and painful. Guilt, anger, sadness, sorrow and grief. On a day when you wish to be celebrating, and sharing the joy of your baby's birth you instead can feel like your world is closing in, threatening to smother you, with many emotions that you struggle to embrace. Friends and family may not understand, after all, you're ok now, right? Trauma leaves its mark and cannot just be wiped away, however much we wish it, and even though months, even years may have passed, the scars can still remain. I have included birthdays in this chapter because many have voiced to me that they have felt this to be a time when they have felt their healing has stalled.

So what can help you when it's your little one's birthday after birth trauma?

All too often we are quick to discount our feelings, we try to put them in a little box, shut down the lid and keep them hidden away. How you feel matters as we saw in a previous chapter. You are important and the day your little one was born, was your day too. It was the day you became a parent, the day when months, even years of dreams and expectations became a reality. When birth is difficult and doesn't go how you had planned it, how that makes you feel matters. Think of it this way. What other traumatic event would anyone go through where they then, every year, were faced with reminders of what they had been through, while at the same time expected to celebrate it? Sadly your dreams and plans may have been shattered, and your start as a new parent, full of anxiety and fear, it's hardly something you would feel like celebrating. Especially so if that day was a day where both you or your baby nearly lost their life.

This was how one mother expressed it. "In all the excitement of present buying, cake baking and balloon blowing there lies lurking in the background a dark oppressive fog. The joy of my child's 3rd birthday is overshadowed by memories and flashbacks of a yesterday that feels all too fresh despite times of advancement. It's been 26,280 hours since my child's birth and most of these hours have passed with some thought, some reliving, deep breathing anxiety that lingers from the point I thought my life was over, that I wouldn't get to know my little girl or grow old with her daddy. It's been 3 years and my daughter is filled with excitement for a day she knows we celebrate. Of course that is only right, I wouldn't wish these thoughts on her so I'll slip on the mask that's showing signs of wear and I'll sing Happy Birthday because that's what you have to do right? The time will come when she's full of cake and happy memories dreaming sweetly in bed, when my mask can be removed and I'll weep for a yesterday that remains so clear in my thoughts, for what it was and for what it could have been."

I can hear you, this is the birth of my baby. You want to be happy, you want to celebrate, but you feel all this pain, and so the feelings of guilt can cascade, tumbling in your mind, causing great distress. As the day approaches you may instead of joy, feel increased anxiety and even fear. The events of the birth may return to your mind, vivid and painful. Everyone around you may be excited and full of expectation, eager to know what you have planned. The guilt that you may not feel the same way can be crushing, and fear can hold you back from telling those who love you how you are really feeling. Guilt that you're finding the birthday of your little one hard can be overwhelming. This isn't how it was supposed to be.

So as you walk your road of recovery what can help when it is the birthday of your little one? Grieving what is lost, how you have been affected and all that this means for you and your family is important. Grieving is part of your healing. Having the space to grieve even this, your child's birthday is vital. It's ok to be sad, to feel hurt, to feel anger and loss. It's ok that for you this day meant trauma and pain. It's ok to struggle and need the love and support, as well as understanding, of those around you. When you have the space to grieve, then guilt as we saw before will start to release its grip.

Take time for yourself! What really helped me was learning, with time, to separate what happened when my daughter was born and the day she came into our world. I realised that I could celebrate her, her life, our happy experiences and memories, the gift that she has been to me, from feelings of pain and hurt that was her birth, where I nearly lost her and my life too. That day was the most terrifying of my life, but also the best day of my life, because it gave me her.

I spent time looking for and dwelling on the tiniest moments of light that I could find in the darkest of hours. One of the things that was a moment of light that I would think about on her birthday was how seconds after her birth they briefly held her above me before they whisked her away, I remembered how she looked, like a tiny fairy, plucked from a flower, a gift I was so grateful to have. It was a precious moment in all the chaos, a moment I could hold on to.

Gradually those moments of light burned brighter and gave me strength and calm. I thought too about all the memories we had built the year before, no matter how small and how precious they were to me, even the difficult days. Then on the day itself, I would try to celebrate those moments, our memories, our survival, our not losing each other. I would however then at the end of the day as she lay sleeping, take time for me. Time to cry, sometimes heartbreaking racking sobs. Time to acknowledge what had been taken from us and how I had been changed. I would let my heart feel it, all of it, knowing that this didn't mean I wasn't celebrating that she was here, or that I loved her.

As the years passed I had time also to reflect on my gratitude to have had a life with her, to watch her grow, take her first step, lose her first tooth, start to walk, start school and many other precious memories. These helped bring me solace.

Never should you feel that you don't matter, your little ones birthday is part of your journey too, your story of becoming a parent and while it may be far from what you had hoped and dreamed it matters.

What about the day itself? Jumping Castles, balloons, cakes, and games. A clown or magician, party bags and gifts. The pressure to have a big celebration can be huge. You can place so much pressure on yourself to do the most amazing birthdays. Remember what really matters. Our children want our time and love. Everything else is extra. So ask. What is right for you, and as a family? What can you reasonably do, and cope with? There are no right or wrongs, birthdays can be as unique as you. Maybe, it's a day out just as a family, or a cosy day in watching films and eating cake. What matters is you are all together. It's important too that you care for yourself, as much as you do for others, and that emotionally you are safe, nurtured and supported. What matters is that your child has you by their side, and can feel the depth of your love. Cakes are eaten, toys get broken, but love lasts forever, and so does building beautiful memories.

It can be helpful to talk with a loved one before the day arrives about what can help to keep you emotionally safe. Ask them to support you in how you would like to spend the day.

Birthdays after birth trauma can be hard. It doesn't mean that you are stalling on your road to healing. Actually, they show the opposite. They show that you are exploring what has happened to you, that you are aware of the emotions that surround you and you are pushing ahead despite the challenges you face.

The future is unwritten

Something that is hard to do after birth trauma is to look to the future. So great is the pain of what has happened and how you have been affected that it can consume the present and leave little in the way of looking forward. I know that for me all I believed the future held was a world where trauma was my companion. I found it hard to plan, I didn't look forward to anything, instead, I felt almost like I was stuck, while everyone around me was enjoying life.

As I started to travel my road, to heal, I began to realise that the future was as yet unwritten. Life is like this book, it has many chapters. Some are wonderful, exciting, full of happiness and joy. Others are like the challenges you face, hard and complex. Just as you can start new chapters, you can also close them. You will still remember what was contained in previous chapters, you may still carry them with you, indeed they may still bring back feelings of hurt, grief or indeed happiness and joy. Yet, you also don't know what the next chapters will bring. I'm sure like me you will try to race ahead, trying to find snippets of what lies there for you. You only though exist in the now, at this moment in time. What will happen next remains unknown, because it hasn't happened….yet.

The truth is that you are the author of your own chapters, your own book. Events will happen, and characters will join you and sometimes leave you, but is you who holds the pen. I know it may not feel that way now. Trauma is telling you that your story, your whole book is about what has happened to you, that you are not safe, that your world is not safe. There are moments while you are healing that you will have to fight that inner narrative. When you will have to fight to take back your life, to believe you will feel safe again, that you are loved and mean everything to those around you. That you are enough in every way and that birth trauma wasn't your fault. You can and you will write a new narrative and new chapters that leads you to your destination.

The future, your future, is unwritten. This is where hope can grow like the snowdrop we mentioned earlier because it means that anything is possible, including recovery. I believed for a very long time I would never recover, and that healing wasn't meant for me. I was looking too far ahead, I was trying to jump my road to the end destination. It felt impossible, too big a leap, too far away. Yet by taking it step by step, it became something within my reach. I took hold of the pen and became the author of my life. I began to write a new chapter that wasn't tainted by trauma's lens and saw life beyond birth trauma. You can too!

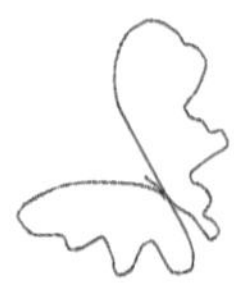

A reflection for you;

- **Hope**. Take your time to look for moments of light both now but also in the past. Let your mind think about the things that made those moments prism light. Was it the strength you showed during a difficult time, was it the feeling you got from a loved one? Reflect on what it shows you about yourself, about what makes you feel happy, loved, and safe. Allow it to show you that hope is strong, that you can feel those ways again. Imagine the light from those moments radiating down from the top of your head, down over your shoulders, down to your chest, your arms, your stomach to your legs. Feel the warmth as it envelopes you, this is hope, this is healing.

- **Recovery**. Look at making a recovery board. You can include things that help you feel calm, things that help you feel supported and loved. You can add songs or quotes, kind things others have said to you or something you may have read. You may wish to make your own affirmations or reminders for when you are feeling difficult emotions. Exercises that help you to feel grounded and secure. Or even create a physical box that contains things to help in times of stress. A favourite book, a picture of a loved one, a special snack, cosy socks, a familiar smell or anything that means calm and safety to you.

- **Growth.** Take some time to think about what is important to you as you navigate healing. What will help you to feel nurtured and supported to grow? Draw a flower with its stem in the soil and open petals. Now write on the soil what helps to nourish you. Then on each of the petals write what you need physically, emotionally, practically and socially to bloom. Maybe your nourishment is rest? Maybe you need to meet with friends to support your social needs. What matters is what supports you. If you are spiritual you could also add this to your petals too.

11

PREGNANCY & BIRTH
A NEW JOURNEY

"Like a butterfly with its wings pinned, trauma holds us in the past never able to move forward until we are healed and set free."

"I always wanted to have a big family, then my son's birth was so traumatic and I thought I could never go through that again."
Jade

With my eyes tightly squeezed shut all I could hear was the bleeping of the machine next to my bed that was tracing my baby's heartbeat. I felt like I was staring death in the face, that I had been given a few extra days, precious extra time with my family and my tiny first daughter. My letters saying goodbye lay in the pocket of my pink hospital bag for when I was gone. It's hard to write to those so precious to you, to put into words how much you love them, knowing that they may be your last sentiments.

My blood pressure was on the rise again so the doctor had decided it was best to induce me to make sure it didn't progress to pre-eclampsia like last time. So here it was, deed day, the day I had been dreading for nine long months. Lucky to cheat death once, I believed fate wouldn't be so kind this time. Did I have hours, maybe days? I had kissed my daughter that morning as we had dropped her off at her nannies and realised it could be the last time I saw her. Her tiny hand had struggled to leave mine and her smile had gripped my heart like a vice when I whispered 'I love you' and said goodbye. Panic, terror, and fear, all gripped me, familiar feelings like every time I left her side, just like the first time she was taken from me.

On the sombre ride to the hospital, I tried to focus my mind, it was two weeks to Christmas but the lights everywhere were off and the morning sky was cold and bleak, I wasn't waiting for Christmas, I felt like I was waiting to see if I would survive this, my baby's birth.

I had always wanted four children but my traumatic birth with my first daughter left me reeling. I felt that there was just no way that I could go through pregnancy and birth again. It was as if the choice had been taken from me, that children would never again bless my life and it was a pain I felt so strongly.

When a birth experience is traumatic it can leave in its wake an intense fear of subsequent pregnancies and births. In fact, sadly many women and/or their partners due to what they have experienced, will feel great anxiety about becoming pregnant again. Indeed some will be so affected that they may feel it impossible to even entertain having another baby, and will take drastic measures to prevent it. Their belief in experiencing a positive birth can feel like holding a beautiful flower and watching it wilt before their eyes. The hopes of expanding their family may feel ripped away.

Other women and/or their partners may feel they have processed and healed from a previous difficult birth experience, however upon finding they are now pregnant again and with an approaching birth, may see a return of difficult memories, confusing feelings and a huge increase in anxiety that they struggle to manage. For some so strong will be their fear due to a previous experience, they may develop what is called secondary 'Tokophobia' which is an intense fear of pregnancy and birth.

Considering a pregnancy and birth after trauma can be scary, or even feel impossible. Yet while it can be challenging, it is possible with the right help and support to heal beyond birth trauma and experience a positive next pregnancy and birth.

I owant another baby

For most couples, the choice to have a baby is usually a happy one and embarked on with much excitement. However if a previous pregnancy or birth has been difficult or traumatic the choice to try for another baby can be thwarted with much anxiety and worry. Previous memories can be overwhelming and even cause them to decide that it just isn't possible. I have heard many times from both women and partners that they really want to have another baby but struggle with how to move beyond their previous experience.

In reality, you don't, which might seem to contradict this whole book which is about healing beyond birth trauma. What I mean however is that each pregnancy and birth is a new and unique experience, it is its own journey and will have its own experiences. Your previous experiences of pregnancy and birth will walk alongside this new journey so to speak. You can't make your previous experience just vanish, nor can you not be affected in some way by what happened before. This is true of many experiences we have in life. You can however find ways to help you in your new experience to both manage the feelings around your previous birth, while also treading this new as yet uncharted journey.

This starts with considering as a couple the possibility of another pregnancy and birth, which will take time and communication. It is important that you are able to openly express your feelings to each other, including your worries and anxieties, and be heard. This can be hard especially if perhaps there is a lack of understanding about how each of you has been affected by the previous experience. It is true also that while you each experienced the birth of your baby, you will have experienced it in very different ways.

Partners often voice to me they have felt helpless, a by-stander who was unable to protect their loved ones. For them, the experience of feeling helpless or unable to prevent the traumatic events can be a heavy weight they carry and they can be worried about how they prevent this from happening again. Women of course are there in the thick of it, the birth happening to them in the physical sense, as well as emotionally. This means their perception is both raw and deep, consideration of that again as we have discussed can be overwhelming.

Openly expressing how you both feel can allow for a deeper understanding of what will be needed to support you both during the next pregnancy and birth. This often leads to a deeper connection as a couple and the ability to see through each other's eyes. This also may mean working through difficult feelings you may have about each other as seen through the trauma lens. Many couples struggle with their relationship after a traumatic birth as we have seen in a previous chapter. It is important that these feelings are resolved as you consider another pregnancy and birth.

It may be that one, or both of you, will need professional support in the form of counselling or therapy with a trained professional. This can be helpful to help understand and deal with the previous trauma before becoming pregnant again. Leaving trauma unresolved can mean a risk of this returning during another pregnancy or birth causing distress, so doing this as part of the preparation for another baby is wise.

Something I hear a lot is the thought of quickly having another birth in order to 'heal' the previous one. This can be thwarted with danger. There is a belief that having a positive birth the next time will somehow make the difficult experience better. Rarely does this seem to be the case, but instead can raise more grief around the previous experience that can cause pain and heartache. Instead, allow time for healing as we have already looked at in previous chapters. Spend time as a couple to talk, understand your feelings, seek help and support. Doing so means you can enter this new journey having acknowledged the effect of your previous experience, while also knowing that you have already made the choice to support this experience to be different. Having support for your previous trauma and talking together as a couple can provide a good foundation on which to consider another pregnancy and birth.

Some hospitals provide birth reflections or debrief sessions that allow you to discuss your previous birth and review your medical notes. These sessions can be helpful in understanding what happened, provide answers to the many questions you may have and also explore if, or what extra support can be put in place in future pregnancies and births to support you physically and emotionally. It is good though to mention again that debriefs of a birth can be hard, often focusing on the medical side and not the emotional impact of your experience. You may find out things that happened that you did not know, which can cause more distress or you may leave not feeling you had the answers you wanted. However, when debriefs are done in a compassionate way they can be supportive of planning and preparing for future pregnancies and births.

So if you are considering another pregnancy after a previous difficult birth it can be good to ask. What can support you if you are considering another baby? What help do you need in your journey of another pregnancy? How can you protect and support your emotional well-being in a future birth? Do you know what will help you feel emotionally safe as individuals and as a couple? Have you given time to healing your previous experience?

Pregnancy after birth Trauma

The line appears, you're pregnant again. You're excited, but pangs of anxiety also grip you making you nervous about the birth. You want another baby, you want to enjoy this pregnancy but the memories of a previous traumatic birth are overwhelming and painful. You sometimes think you can't do this or give birth again.

Due to the circumstances of your previous pregnancy and/or birth, you might be feeling anxious, unsafe, and vulnerable both physically and/or emotionally. What can support you during this new pregnancy?

Connect with your partner. Communication is vital and you will need to support each other. Talk about how you feel and what you both need for this pregnancy. Be open about your worries and needs for this new journey. Provide emotional space and safety for each other. Try to attend appointments together and ask questions of those who are over your care. Complete your birth plan together and also have frank discussions about how you can advocate for your birth choices. It is so important that each of you is open and honest with each other. There can be a tendency to want to protect the other person and not 'add' to their already existing anxiety. However, this only can cause more issues, misunderstandings and distrust. Make sure that when it comes to the birth, both of you are fully aware of what you are happy to accept, and what you don't want to happen and can advocate for this. I always encourage couples to sit together and make a plan for their birth that covers different scenarios so they feel prepared and aware of each other's needs should they arise.

Research. Try to spend some time researching what can support you in your pregnancy and birth. What your choices are, what and how to support you physiologically and emotionally. Look at evidence-based information to help you make informed choices about your care, then share this with your care providers.

Consider what things can help you feel emotionally safe this time. If there was a particular element of your birth that you found hard, such as an intervention, research what can help to prevent it, what choices there are around it or what may be alternatives. Arm yourself with as much information as you can. Allow this to support you to advocate for yourself and your needs.

Decide what is right for you. Each birth is individual. What you need to support this pregnancy and birth to be positive will be unique to you. Listen to your instincts, consider the evidence, talk to your healthcare provider and explore what you need. It may be a care-plan that supports you to have a physiological birth, or it may be a well-planned elective caesarean section. What matters is having the birth that is right for you. Making a personal birthing plan that includes your wishes can be supportive to both you and your birth partner as well as those caring for you. You can include in your plan things that may be triggers for you, or aspects of care that you definitely do not want. Things you want your birth partner to advocate for you, or things you need those around you to be aware of.

Remember this is about you being supported, so include things in your plan that underpin this. This plan should be about emotional safety, not just the medical side of your birth. What matters is that these are what is right for you. When I have supported couples to make these plans it can be surprising what comes out. It can also serve as a good way to explore your choices if you feel unsure about certain aspects of your care.

Seek Support. Be honest and open with those who are caring for you about what this new journey requires from them. Explain that you are anxious due to your previous experience and ask what they can offer to help you. Find healthcare professionals who will support you, respect your choices and respect the birth that you desire. Surround yourself with those who will work with you and acknowledge the experience of your previous birth, instead of minimising it, and encourage you on this new journey. Do not be afraid to say No if you are not happy with any plans advised. Also, ask for second opinions or to change a caregiver if you are not feeling supported.

Ask for help from family and friends. Explain how you are feeling and that their understanding and support will help you on this journey. Trust them to hold you, to be there on days that are hard, to advocate and protect you.

Some hospitals have specialist midwives and services that support women after previous difficult maternity journeys. Ask if these are available for you. Other areas may provide extra support through perinatal/maternal mental health services or charities, again ask if these can be available to support you.

Find the strengths of your previous birth. Even in the most difficult of experiences, there are strengths that can be found. Exploring this and finding these can help support you in your next birth. This can be done with your partner, a doula or in a supportive birthing community.

These strengths can be knowing that this time you have more awareness, you know your body more, what your limits are and what your needs are. You also know what works for you, what things are important to you and what you don't want to happen this time. You are taking with you into this journey way more knowledge about yourself and the birth experience. Try to reframe things you experienced to see that they can give insight into how things can be supported to be better this time and what you need to attain it. Then communicate this to those around you.

Make a birthing support plan. A birthing support plan that includes your wishes, needs, wants and don't wants, can be supportive both to you and those caring for you. This can be done with your partner and include their wishes too. You may include things that you wish for should your plans change, or considerations of interventions that you may or may not wish to have.

Keep it brief and readable for those who will need to see it. Your birthing support guide should be realistic for you and your care providers but also include the emotional support you need. As mentioned before some hospitals have specialist midwives and obstetricians that work with women and their partners who have experienced a previous traumatic birth and will complete a birth plan with you. Ask at your antenatal booking appointment if this is possible for you. Any plan you complete should be trauma-informed namely it takes into consideration your previous experiences and this then should be used to inform your planned care going forward.

The one I like to share with couples is the 'Birth Tree', the trunk of the tree is for the things that you wish for your birth. The branches can be used for the things you don't want or smaller plans for if things change such as if an induction of labour is recommended. There are many types of plans you can use, so find one that works for you and reflects your needs. Also include in your plan the practical side such as who will care for any other children you have, who will be your birth partners, what you need for your labour and who will support you in the postnatal period.

Things may change. Even when you do all you can to support your birth to be better this time this doesn't mean that things can't change. Having various options and knowing what choices are there to support you can allow you to manage any change that may occur. Planning for a few different situations can help you feel in control and reduce anxiety. Remember that some things are out of your control, and this can make you feel vulnerable, but there are also many things you can plan for using your knowledge of your previous experience and all your newly acquired information.

Find your advocate. During your birth have someone with you that can advocate for your wishes. This may be your partner, family member, or friend. Some couples will hire a doula or birth worker or you may have support via a midwife or other healthcare professional/service. In your pregnancy have frank open discussions about what your wishes are and ask how they can support you. You can even practice how they can advocate for you in different situations. Also, find support from a community that reflects your wishes. This may be a home birth group, a caesarean section support group or other supportive birth group. Peer support is powerful, it can help you to feel confident and understood in your choices.

Be kind to yourself. Recognise and acknowledge that you may hold beliefs that can have an impact on this birth. Your previous experience may make you believe you need 'to be perfect' or that you are 'not good enough' or that your previous experience was 'your fault'. Challenge these beliefs and build new ones, we discussed this in previous chapters.

Don't expect too much of yourself or let any bad days cause you to doubt your new journey. Remember that feeling anxious or worried is valid and while this may walk with you, you are already finding ways to make it different this time. Do not let others cause you to doubt yourself or your choices in what is right for you. Be mindful of expectations both you may place on yourself and allow from others. Try to talk to yourself as you would a dear friend. Show yourself compassion, forgiveness and love.

Calming strategies. Finding ways to help you feel calm and in control is important. Using deep breathing, mindfulness, grounding techniques or visualisation are some of the ways to support you emotionally. Find what works for you! Mindfulness can be helpful as it brings us back to the now, leaving the past and the future where is it. Mindfulness can be anything from a walk in nature to yoga or meditation, or just listening to your favourite music. These can be used to manage feeling anxious during your pregnancy and also during the birth itself. Another thing that can be calming is spending time connecting with your baby. Talk, sing or just focus on your baby. Imagine what they may look like or what your hopes will be for them.

Find your affirmation. This may sound cheesy but having a saying that is personal to you can be helpful in times of anxiety. Find an affirmation that gives you hope, that provides you with grounding and helps to bring in calm thoughts. Your affirmation is personal to you and as unique as you are. You can record it either in your voice or your partner's to play during pregnancy and labour. An example of an affirmation is 'I am safe'. It could be an encouraging saying you have heard or even a funny antidote. I will be honest here and say I did struggle with this myself. Then I found 'wet noodle'. I can see your perplexed look! I would say this over and over to myself and imagine I was a noodle, floppy and free, plain and untroubled. I've no idea why this works for me but it does and always makes me smile. My anxiety just seems to float away!

Believe that a positive birth is possible for you. One of the hardest things to do following a traumatic birth is to believe that a positive birth is possible. When trust is broken, we feel hurt, anger and disappointment. It is possible to be emotionally supported to have a birth that can be a healing experience. Remember that each pregnancy and birth is different, that you are different, but also that you are more aware of your needs and wishes. A positive birth experience is unique to each person. Being able to put in place a birthing support plan to help you and the right care can give you the confidence and belief that it is possible.

Also, tell yourself regularly that it is possible and rely on those around you to help make this a possibility. If you find that you wish to birth a certain way and this isn't being supported then ask again, request to see someone else till you do find the support you need. Just remember that often it is the little things that matter. Just because you have a caesarean section doesn't mean you can't still have soft music or skin-to-skin with your new baby. While you may find that some of your medical needs limit your choices there is much you still can choose. Regardless of how you decide to give birth, there are things you can do to make it positive, the biggest of all of these is knowing that you matter and so do your needs.

Balance it out. Nothing is going to completely remove the anxiety and worry you will feel and I'm not going to lie and tell you otherwise. I do believe however you can help to balance it out. Imagine one of those old scales with the two hanging brass bowls. On one side is all the worry and fear and anxiety, on the other side fill the bowl with things that are positive and bring you hope. It may be your birth plan, support of family, or happy things about this pregnancy journey such as your scan pictures. Try keeping a journal of your hopes, imagining your baby and what it may look like. It can be anything that fills your bowl, but let it help balance out the fear so it is manageable. On days when the worry and fear seem too much have in place things that help you to cope. Go for a walk, reach out to friends and family, and do things to help you feel connected to your baby. In reality, the scales may feel heavy to the side of anxiety and this is completely understandable, but finding balance is possible and can help you manage till you hold your baby in your arms.

Pregnancy and birth after suffering a previous traumatic experience can be daunting in so many ways. I have supported so many families over the years to have a birth experience that has kept them emotionally safe, as well as physically safe. I believe that this can be possible for you too with the right help and support as you heal beyond birth trauma.

I heard her cry as she was lifted onto my tummy. I was ok and so was she. Over the next few hours, she never left my side and it felt beyond surreal. This was how it was meant to be and I felt a pang of pain as I realised what I had lost with my first. Then tiny footsteps, wide eyes full of wonder and a big smile appeared from around the curtain. My daughter was a big sister now and it was time to go home. As we drove home the light was almost gone and everywhere there were twinkling lights filling windows and adorning trees, I closed my eyes and sighed with sheer relief. I had survived, we both had and I was the most grateful person on earth. I took my tiny daughter's hand in mine and gripped it so tight as we carried our new baby, into our home.

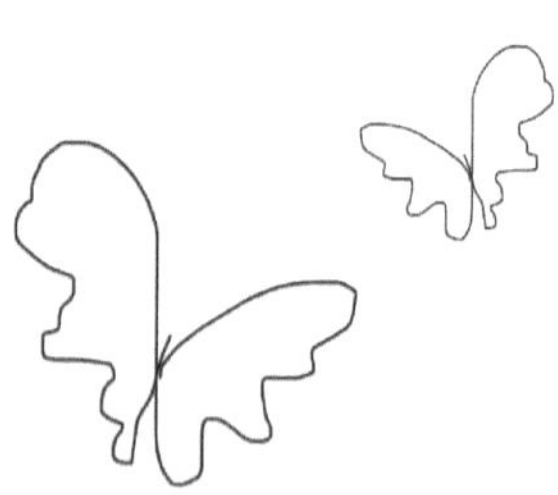

12

THE JOURNEY OF NEONATAL

"The first time ever I saw your face I thought the sun rose in your eyes, and the moon and the stars were the gifts you gave to the dark and the endless skies."
Roberta Flack

"For me, my birth trauma was seeing my baby fight for her life when she was born at just 27 weeks."
Alison

They held you above me for the briefest of moments and then they took you away, you made the tiniest cry, so weak, such a struggle. Then you were gone and I felt like you were a million miles away. I closed my eyes to shut out the words and the chaos that surrounded me and tried to remember your face.

Tears stung my eyes because I didn't know if I would see you again and pain gripped my heart tearing it in two. Then there were bright lights and white walls, masked people all around me, falling, then darkness took me captive and try as I might I couldn't remember your face.'

There are no words to describe the first time you see your baby. For nine months you wonder and try to picture the life growing inside you. What colour eyes they may have, if they will have hair and if they will inherit the tiny dimple you inherited from your mother and her mother before.

When your baby is born and all has gone well with your birth, you are handed your baby to hold and you get to know every detail, every finger, every toe. You breathe in their smell and stroke their face and love for your baby envelopes you like an enchanting spell. But when your baby is born early or if there are complications during birth and they need to be cared for in the neonatal unit, you may not get to hold your baby for hours, days and sometimes weeks. The emotional impact on you can be enormous and long-lasting. The guilt of not holding or being able to be with your baby in those early hours and days can weigh heavy on your heart for many weeks, or months after, sadly sometimes even years.

When my daughter was born six weeks early she was taken from me to the resuscitation cot and it felt like a lifetime before her cry pierced the room. The midwife held her above me for a few seconds and then she was gone, taken to the neonatal unit to be cared for. I was then worked on by the medical team for a retained placenta before being rushed to the theatre to save my life. As I was whisked down the corridors all I could see was the blinding bright lights on the ceiling, so I closed my eyes and tried to picture my daughter's face, but I couldn't. I believed I was going to die and I would never get to know what she looked like, if she had any hair, what colour her eyes were and if she looked anything like me. I didn't even know how much she weighed.

It was almost 24 hours after her birth before I finally got to see my daughter for the first time. When I was finally well enough to be moved to the postnatal ward the arduous journey to neonatal to see her every day began. Once I was well enough to be discharged the pain of being sent home without her was so overwhelming.

The room is dark and my pillow is wet with silent tears. I desperately need the nourishment of sleep, but it has escaped me. I wish the hours away waiting for the light of day to return and cast its glow upon the earth once again. Unable to bear the silence of the dark any longer I raise my battered body to sit on the edge of the bed. There is no baby's cry to pierce the night, no baby's skin soft and warm to stroke. No baby to relieve my aching breasts full of milk. The pain in my body is nothing compared to the pain in my heart. I'm home but my baby is lying in neonatal without me, and my arms ache to hold her. So as the darkness starts to give way to dawn, I drive the few miles to the hospital, it feels like a lifetime, every red light prolonging the agony till I'm with my baby again.

If I could run to neonatal I would, but instead, I stumble there, every step takes so much effort, but I manage it. The staff seem surprised I'm there so early but I know I won't be leaving her again. I look at her lying there in her incubator, tubes and cannulas everywhere, her feet black from all the heel prick tests and I feel so much guilt. The days I was in HDU she lay here alone, had anyone comforted her when she cried, had she been scared and in pain? What did she feel when having her phototherapy, needles and drugs, did she cry for me wondering where her mummy was?

The pain I feel are like stabs to my heart. But I'm here now to hold and protect her. She is mine and I love her with every inch of my being, that love has a hold on my heart and is scary and overwhelming all at once.

The birth had nearly killed us both, robbed me of her, and her of me. At 34 weeks she had been taken from me and started her life, her first hours and days alone, but no more. I would be here, no matter what it took, no matter how long, because she was mine.

So for weeks, the neonatal unit became my life and my home, I slept in a chair by my daughter's side every night just wanting to be with her. While I had been an in-patient my days had consisted of wheeling myself down to the unit in a wheelchair and then sitting by her incubator helpless. I was so ill that it took everything I had to manage to stay with her as long as I could. I would watch the nurses clean her, change her, and feed her in the plastic box that was her home, which felt like a wall keeping her from me. The machines constantly bleeped and alarms signalled for a nurse to attend, more drugs given and wires covered her tiny body monitoring her heart, her breathing, everything. She needed phototherapy and so for hours, the light would cover her skin, her tiny body fighting to flush the jaundice out. My time holding her was fleeting and I would return to the ward empty handed listening to the cries of the other babies and I would cry myself to sleep. The vision of her in my head kept me going, kept me fighting to stay alive. Every time I saw her laying in her incubator I marvelled that she was really mine because she was like a fairy that had lost her wings and had been given to me to love.

The unit was a scary place and I felt out of my depth. The machines beeped and buzzed and I was terrified to touch her. I felt so inexperienced and unsure as a mother. I had never experienced anything like this. Around me other babies clung to life, some so tiny it was hard to see them under the equipment that was keeping them alive. My well-being was lost in just coping each day. I wasn't sure if or when I ate and sleep came in minutes not hours. Emotionally I was as battered and bruised as my physical body. I felt like I was walking in a horrible nightmare from which I couldn't wake up.

When finally she was well enough to be moved to a cot I felt less separated from her, I could reach and touch her without having to ask but I still felt scared to just pick up my own baby, she was so small and I worried about the tubes and cannulas. Slowly I gained the confidence to pick her up on my own and I just couldn't get enough. It made my heart soar just to hold her whenever I wanted and check every detail of her. Her pointy elf ears and tiny nose. I could not believe how tiny she was and yet so perfect like a dream. I was intoxicated by her smell and felt a love that invaded my soul, crept and flowed through my veins, and I was never going to let go. When I did have to let go when she went back in her cot and my arms were left empty it felt like physical pain. I felt like I was finally getting to know her, my baby that had grown inside me for only 34 weeks before she came into the world. I still remember those precious moments like the greatest gifts the universe could give me and it felt like time was standing still.

The journey of neonatal didn't end though when finally we came home. While the relief to be out of the unit and in my own home was huge, our experience had changed me. Everything felt different, I felt scared and on high alert. I had an overwhelming need to protect my tiny daughter, and this made me anxious beyond measure. While the rest of the world was moving on, I felt stuck. I was still feeling the effects of our traumatic experience, and yet I didn't understand what was happening. All I knew was that the world had changed, I had changed, I felt scared and alone. The responsibility of caring for this tiny human that I had nearly lost was overwhelming. My physical recovery was slow and the fear that I would still die was very real. No one had prepared me for this, the cascading of emotions, the fear and uncertainty. I felt like everything we had been through suddenly hit me like a brick wall and I had no idea how to find peace again.

So it's true to say that having a baby in a neonatal unit is a difficult journey. To give birth and have your baby taken from you sometimes without you even seeing them is so distressing. It may be hours or even days before you can see your baby and for babies born very early, it can be weeks before you may even be able to hold them. Suddenly instead of you caring for your new baby, the care is taken over by nurses and doctors. Each day is difficult as you navigate the many challenges of having a premature/sick baby. In some cases every day your baby is battling just to survive. Going home each day without your baby is heartbreaking. This isn't how it was supposed to be.

Plastic boxes

You stare through the plastic, in amongst the wires that seem to be everywhere, is your tiny baby. The beep of the machines is constant and relentless, and every so often an alarm sounds making your heart beat faster as you jump to your feet to check your baby is ok.

Nurses come and go sometimes opening the portholes to attend to your baby's needs. Every day as you make your way to the unit you wonder and worry what that day will bring. This tiny life that once was inside you is now in the big wide world, maybe too soon, and now you patiently wait each day while others keep your baby alive.

While in neonatal you can often go into coping mode. It can leave you with intense feelings of sadness, grief, guilt, shame, anger, disbelief and numbness, a rollercoaster that takes you for a ride each day. It can be especially difficult when your baby suffers medical setbacks and you hold your breath as you wait to see what will happen. Having a baby in the neonatal unit may be one of the most stressful times you ever experience.

The challenges of neonatal are many. Parents struggle with the separation from their baby, bonding can be an issue and some feel that their baby doesn't feel like theirs. Having to go home each day and leave your baby can have a massive emotional impact. Feeling a sense of having no control can also be difficult to cope with, parents can feel that they have no say or that they are not involved in caring for their baby.

Being in a constant state of worry and threat for days or weeks on end can have a profound effect on emotional well-being. Life in the neonatal unit is constantly up and down, with good and bad days. Parents can feel like their life is on hold and doing normal daily activities becomes virtually impossible. Many partners find they have to return to work, meaning new mothers are left to visit the unit alone or rely on family and friends for help and support.

Feelings of guilt can be strong. There can be guilt over the birth, why their baby was born early and if they could have prevented it. Guilt for not being able to be with their baby all the time, especially if there are other children to care for and guilt for feeling exhausted both emotionally and physically while wanting to do everything they can for their babies. Some may even struggle to visit their baby due to finding the unit itself an overwhelming environment or seeing their baby so unwell deeply traumatic. Of course, some babies born early may require many months in a neonatal unit but the outside world doesn't stop. Trying to juggle family life with a baby in neonatal can be challenging, to say the least.

There is also a sense of loss and grief. Grieving the loss of the end of a pregnancy, a wanted birth experience, the early days with a new baby, establishing feeding and intimate time bonding as a family. This isn't how anyone ever dreamed of welcoming a new baby into the world.

For some families, there are the added difficulties of coming to terms with long-term physical or medical complications in their premature baby. The reality of how life has now changed and the impact on the whole family can be overwhelming.

It is little surprise then that many parents will recall the journey of neonatal as being traumatic with some sadly going on to develop PTSD. Whether a stay in neonatal is long or short the emotional effects can be long-lasting.

Going Home

Taking home your baby after any time in a neonatal unit is filled with many emotions. Happiness that finally you can take your little one home, as well as relief, is more than words can express. But along with the joy can be fear and worry.

After months of being in a unit with staff supporting your baby 24/7, being solely responsible for their care can be daunting. There has always been someone close by to ask advice and rely on, plus alarms and machines to reassure you all is ok, but now it is just you, scared, worried anxious, parents.

Your neonatal baby has lots to adjust to in their new environment called home. There are different sights, sounds, smells and temperatures, and even the lighting is different. Sometimes all these changes can be very overwhelming for your baby. This can result in a very unsettled baby and very anxious parents. Getting to grips with feeding, sleep and caring for your baby is a huge transition and takes time. If your baby has continuing health issues or medical needs this too is stressful to manage and adjust to. It is true also that often parents voice that the true impact of the time they spent on the unit with their baby only fully hit them once they went home. Emotionally this can take a heavy toll on new parents as they struggle to adjust to life with their baby and also juggle feelings that are overwhelming. Yes, the neonatal journey doesn't end when you leave the unit but can continue for many months or years.

Of course, sadly not all families will get to take their precious babies home. The devastation is beyond measure and specialist help is vital for those who lose their babies. I know that many families have voiced to me that after their loss and going home with empty arms, they have been offered little in the way of support. As a result, trauma can take hold adding to the pain and heartache these families already carry.

If you are a family that has lost your baby you're not alone and there are others that understand how you are feeling. It is hard but reach out for the support you need. There are many national organisations that offer information and support as well as peer support from others who have experienced such deep loss too.

From me personally, I want you to know that your baby mattered and their life mattered, however short. They will always be part of you and part of your family. While their time with you may have been short they have brought so much love to your heart and you will carry them with you always.

Finding Support

Sometimes birth trauma is because of the journey of neonatal. It was definitely a contributing part of mine and lingered with me for a very long time. While so much focus is on the baby and understandably so, parents need care too, especially emotionally. Supporting parents with the difficult emotions of a neonatal journey can help to reduce trauma.

If you have had a baby on the neonatal unit what can help you with the feelings you may have about your experience?

There are many wonderful organisations that provide support for families that offer both online support but also phone lines and support groups. Ask your unit for any information they may have on support local to you. Some neonatal units have on-site counselling services for you to access so that you can be supported emotionally while you navigate this difficult time, this may be via peer support or dedicated psychological therapies.

When you go home with your baby again ask about what support is available. This can vary in each area, some have outreach programs to support you when your baby is discharged. Others have neonatal nurses that will visit you at home to provide additional support. Some areas run support groups for you to attend to meet other parents who also have had the journey of neonatal. There are also national support groups that can help you connect to other parents.

It may however take weeks, even months for you to feel the full impact of what you have been through. Processing the experience of neonatal can take time and as we said before often parents report feeling like they suddenly hit a wall months later which can lead to a re-surfacing of many emotions. Those around you with good intentions may try to help by reassuring you that everything is ok now or your baby is healthy and doing well. While this may be true it may not mean you are not struggling. If you find that you are troubled by your experience, having feelings of guilt, anger or sadness or feeling you are traumatised or experiencing symptoms of PTSD then accessing help and support is important. What else can you do?

TALK to someone you feel comfortable with about your feelings such as your partner, family, GP, health visitor or community neonatal nurse.

REACH OUT for support or ask for local support groups. There are also many online support pages for parents of premature babies and talking to others who have been through a similar experience can help greatly.

Finding others who too have been through the journey of neonatal can bring companionship and solace.

BE GENTLE with yourself and remember you have been through a very difficult time. Allow yourself the space to process your time in the neonatal unit. Don't expect too much of either yourself or your baby. Time bonding with your baby and finding your way as a parent is important and this will take time.

ASK for help from family and friends even in practical ways. They may not fully understand your feelings around your time in neonatal with your baby, but they will be eager to help in any way they can.

REMEMBER your feelings are part of processing your experience. You may feel worried, scared and overwhelmed but also anger, grief and loss. Counselling can help you manage your feelings and help you understand and work through them so that they do not progress to the point where they overwhelm you.

We cannot prevent babies from coming into the world early or sometimes the traumatic events that may surround their birth or their time in neonatal. I personally know the toll having a baby in the neonatal unit can take and how this can stay with you. I have also supported many families over the years who have had a baby in the neonatal unit and have heard from them about the many ways in which they have been affected. Just like with other forms of birth trauma this can be as unique as the person.

I believe that every family deserves to have the emotional support they need as they navigate the challenges that come with a baby born early or sick. I'm passionate that this should be offered routinely and available both on the unit and once families go home. There is still much to do in this regard but I have definitely seen much improvement over the years and I hope the emotional impact continues to be acknowledged and researched. I also believe that it is vital families are at the centre of neonatal services, and that they are listened to and regarded as equals in the care of their babies. For me, a lot of what I found traumatic could have been prevented by simple communication, emotional support and help to care for my baby while on the unit.

If the journey of neonatal has been part of your story then know that it matters, that your feelings need the time and space to be understood, acknowledged and then supported to heal. I look back on the time my daughter and I spent in neonatal and there is a mix of emotions. I still feel some sadness and loss, pain that my own needs were so ignored, that no one prepared me or offered support for everything we had been through. I also see those moments of light, the strength I saw in my tiny daughter, and how she inspired me to find my own strength. The memories of watching her overcome being born early, to doing things they said she may not, to battling challenges that frustrated us both, to coping with some of the lasting legacy of neonatal. As a young woman now I cherish those memories and in truth, she will always be, my tiny, fairy baby.

Yes with help and support you can navigate the journey of neonatal and the months and years that follow taking your beautiful baby home.

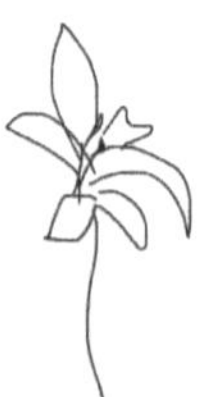

13

HOW CAN WE PREVENT BIRTH TRAUMA?

"Listening is a magnetic and strange thing, a creative force. When we are listened to it creates, makes us unfold and expand."
Karl A. Menninger

"I know that my trauma was something that could have been avoided and that is the most painful aspect of it all."
Ruth

I long for the day when pregnancy and birth are no longer a traumatic experience for anyone. The reality is that this still feels a long way off. However, I believe that there is much we can do as healthcare services, society and individuals to prevent families from feeling traumatised by their maternity and birth experiences. This is what this chapter covers.

Over the years as I have sought to accept and share my story I have struggled to come to terms with how some have reacted to it, and me as the person sharing it. I honestly believed that anyone who heard my journey of birth trauma would be horrified and would want to understand it so that lessons could be learnt on how we could prevent it from happening again. Sadly this hasn't always been the case and while there have been many who have listened, there have been just as many who have surprised me by their reluctance to hear, acknowledge and support not only my story but many of the families I've supported since.

I have pondered the reason for this over a long time as I believe it is a key barrier to improving services and preventing birth from being traumatic. We hear all the time that women feel they weren't listened to, or have felt dismissed during their birth and in reality, I think this is even more true when birth has been traumatic. So why is it so difficult to acknowledge that birth is sometimes traumatic?

We have already said before that birth should be a happy time, the bringing of new life into a family, so when this isn't the case it can be hard to explore why. When women or new parents are struggling with their mental health due to perhaps a health condition, the challenges of being a new parent or because of social or economic situations this is largely acknowledged and understood but also mostly free of a source of blame. We can readily accept that parenthood brings challenges that affect our emotional well-being. We also accept and have much more awareness around general mental health conditions and how this can be impacted by the parenting journey. There also have been good steps forward in offering perinatal mental health services, yet what about the maternity journey itself?

When families voice however that they are struggling with their mental health due to a difficult birth experience there can be a reluctance to accept this. We may ask why and from my experience the reasons can be complex, some being not having an understanding of what birth trauma is, then not being sure how to offer support. Sadly though over the years, it has become more evident to me that a large portion of trauma caused at birth is a result of poor care or damage to a mother and/or her baby and this has been evident from several reports and investigations conducted into maternity units. This of course then raises the question of who or what is to blame.

For those who care for families during a maternity journey, it can be hard to acknowledge that poor care has been the reason for some families feeling traumatised. Not wishing to face the reality that care has been lacking, it can be easier to dismiss the voice of those who share how they have been affected. It is almost like if it isn't spoken or heard then it hasn't happened. It can be true also that it can be viewed as a rare event of an unfortunate few.

Over the years the reasons why improvement in maternity seems such a hard thing to attain has always puzzled me. I believe that many of the issues that women tell us cause them to feel traumatised are the same as those that were echoed years ago. So if we know what they are and we are having the same conversations about how women and families need to be listened to, why has change been hard to achieve?

I do not believe that inherently anyone truly comes to the birth space to cause harm to families. Yet this can be the result when there is a loss of understanding of personal intent versus personal impact. I have worked, and am friends with many who work in maternity services, no one would disagree with the challenges faced by anyone who supports families on the maternity journey. Many staff voice that the system itself impacts the care given and is the cause of much of the trauma experienced by families. While this is true in some aspects, there must be an acknowledgement of the personal responsibility needed to offer good care. The healthcare system is flawed in places and the pressures are high as a result but there is more to consider as to why many birth experiences are causing harm to families.

One thing that has stood out to me over and over again is the perception of the roles of maternity staff by others and also by themselves. I have talked to and observed many different individuals and opinions over the years I have been involved in maternity improvement at local and national levels. What has always struck me is how identity is such a key part of the roles in maternity, and how this has sadly caused some to lose sight of the reality of birth from the family's point of view. It can be the case that birth becomes more about the person giving the care and the experience they believe should happen or they themselves wish to have, than the person who is actually giving birth. Let me illustrate.

Once in deep conversation with a midwife, she lost herself telling me of her experiences in her role and the privilege she felt to be a 'bringer of life to the world', of the euphoria she felt handing a new baby to its parents. It was interesting to me how sadness fell upon her as she told me she felt this was taken away from her once the birth became more medical or interventions were needed requiring the added support of a wider team. This was echoed by others in similar ways and I reflected on this for a long time. I couldn't help but question the importance of the birth experience and who this mattered most to the caregiver, or the woman, her baby and her family.

While it may be true that it is a wonderful thing to share the birthing space with a family, surely it is their experience and what they need that should matter. No one can question what a privilege it is to support families with the birth of their baby but in that birthing room where there is a sharing of a special intimate space, it should never be about any individual's personal thoughts, ideas or wishes but only that family and their needs. Yet what happens when personal identity, belief or view of how birth should be, pervades the birthing space?

The elephant in the room

When I reflect on improving birth for families it reminds me of an ancient parable about a group of blind men who having never come across an elephant before seek to learn about this magnificent animal by touch. Each man feels a different part of the elephant's body, such as a tusk or a leg, and then explains it to the others. Of course, each man's description is so different from the other that they are in complete disagreement on what this creature could be. As a result, much debate and arguments result, each man claiming to be right and the others wrong.

The point of the parable is to highlight that we all have the tendency to base our 'truth' on our own experiences, while often ignoring other people's experiences, coming to conclusions based on our own thoughts and beliefs.

The parable goes on to explain that the men, after much disagreement eventually stop talking and instead start listening to each, collaborating in order to 'see' the whole elephant. In time the men realise that they were all partially right, and all partially wrong. Why? Because our subjective experience may not be the totality of the truth. This teaches us that while an experience or a belief can be true for us, this isn't always the case for others. It shows us the need to evaluate when there may be a lack of information available to us and also the need to respect and consider different perspectives. True listening involves putting aside our views, to consider the views of others.

I love this parable because it always makes me think about pregnancy and birth. We all know that birth is physiologically within the ability of women and that it can be a powerful and positive experience. There is some evidence to suggest that certain circumstances and environmental factors support birth to be possible without intervention and a positive experience for all in attendance. It could be that this is our subjective experience or it may be that this is what we believe from the information we have been presented with. This may include where or how a woman should birth, it may include the way pain in birth can be managed or supported and how this can impact the woman and her baby. It may be what the physiological norm is for the birth process. This 'truth' that we may have experienced or come to understand or believe can mean us seeing birth a certain way.

However, this isn't the absolute truth. We know that the birth experience is complex and different for each woman. This can cause difficulties when looking to improve services or provide care that families really need. It requires those who offer the choices around birth, to see the whole truth not just one truth that may be shaped by their own perceptions of how they feel birth should be.

Each family is an individual with different needs. These needs will be shaped by previous experiences, culture, personal beliefs and circumstances. Some families are struggling with economic hardships, social issues, and physical or mental health conditions. There are also many inequalities that impact on maternity journeys. This all can alter how they view what they need to support them in their pregnancy and birth.

A family's truth or perspective in current pregnancies and birth will also be affected by previous maternity experiences. It may be that a previous pregnancy or birth was traumatic, or that they lost a baby. Maybe they have endured many miscarriages or the long journey of fertility treatment. Maybe they were given poor care and so have broken trust in healthcare professionals. So the perspective they may hold on birth can be completely different, even from what they may have thought before.

While evidence and information can offer some perspectives, there is also the human side, the person and family at the centre who will bring complexity to the birth experience that needs to be considered.

So what can we learn from the parable of the blind men and the elephant?

That when it comes to pregnancy and birth sometimes we need to stop talking and instead listen. While we have many forms of evidence and reports on which to draw our 'truth', as well as our own experiences, we need to listen to families and what they are voicing about their individual needs. Hearing their perspective can be powerful, it allows us to gain a full picture, a reality of them and their circumstances. It also allows for individualised, trauma-informed care. Sometimes what we may see as a priority is far from what the person actually needs. We will only know this by listening to their perspective.

Even when there may be evidence that supports an aspect of maternity care that seems to be a whole truth is it?

For a family considering any choices they make they have to be able to make a choice that reflects them as a whole. While reports or evidence may give knowledge that is one 'truth' a family may have a very different view of the choices they wish to make. Any choices we make always come with consequences, so sometimes families need to be able to live with those choices in the future. This means they may make choices that to us feel uncomfortable. While we can share the knowledge, or as in the case of the parable, the part of the elephant we have examined, we need to also hear other perspectives to form a whole picture. Sadly it can be the case that certain recommendations for birth are put forth as the right choice to families, without an understanding of their actual circumstances and needs. It doesn't matter how evidence-based something is, if it isn't right for that individual great harm can be caused especially emotionally by coercing women into things that are not right for them. There needs to be the seeing of the whole picture as it were, this involves time but also the putting aside of personal beliefs and opinions so consideration can be given to finding approaches that support the safety of mothers and babies. This can be especially hard if it feels like this is a negative reflection on someone's personal identity.

To illustrate this I have over the years supported many families who have sadly lost their babies during birth. The grief and pain are unimaginable and as a result, a subsequent pregnancy is full of fear and anxiety. For many the need for reassurance, both by medical checks and a robust birth plan are important in managing their concerns. Many have wished for what some would think of as a very medicalised birth, even in some cases a planned caesarean section to support the reduction of triggers and the safe arrival of their baby. Countless times I have seen families' concerns dismissed, their wishes refused and as a result, they have had to battle for the choices and care they need. This only causes more stress and harm to women and their babies. The evidence may say that the chances of loss again are low, or that there are no actual medical reasons for that woman to have a caesarean section. But what about her emotional needs, what about the protection of her mental health on this maternity journey?

Care that is trauma-informed and supportive of mental health takes into consideration the whole picture. It doesn't dismiss but instead listens, hears and considers the human side. It allows for the provision of individualised care that keeps women safe emotionally as well as medically. Which brings me next to, are we really listening?

Are we really listening?

When we think about prevention of trauma during the maternity journey we have to be able to hear, with a view to seeing where change is needed. In the many years that I have supported women after traumatic births one clear theme is constant, that women feel they are not listened to, both in antenatal care and also during birth and the postnatal period. Listening to the concerns, experiences and perspectives of women and families is vital. Without doing so we will never prevent birth from being traumatic.

We also need to collaborate to see the whole 'truth' which includes not only another person's perspective but also their needs. If a woman suffers from anxiety she may need the reassurance of a maternity ward, or, she may need the comforts of her own home, each is valid. The choice should be available for what is right for her, in her circumstances, and then support given for those choices as much as possible. This can be especially challenging if a woman is considered 'high risk' which can often limit choice. Choice however is important, it can give back a sense of control, help women feel involved in their care and allow for a more positive experience. So what if that choice challenges our personal view of how birth should be?

We need to see that no one is truly right, no one is truly wrong. Each viewpoint has much to add to the conversation. Yet, women have the right to say what will happen to them, their bodies and their babies. When we shut down choice, when we mandate how women should birth we risk causing great harm.

This applies too when looking at improving or developing maternity services. We need to see the whole truth and other perspectives. Engagement with those who need maternity services gives a fuller understanding of what birth is to each family. This can be hard however because it may mean hearing things that are painful or create uncomfortable feelings. Engagement only works if the aim is to truly listen with the intent to hear and then take action. We need to remember that each personal experience brings with it much that we can learn both positive and what needs to improve, both are important. Rather than let our subjective experience, or limited information become our whole truth, let us listen, work together and see the many perspectives that others can offer so we can continue to support birth for everyone.

Some in maternity services have voiced that they have felt their role or personal identity has been attacked, this is where personal reflection is so important and where we need to listen even more. We may need to seek to understand why hearing the perspectives of others is difficult for us, why this feels like a personal attack and if this is preventing us from seeing the whole picture. Doing this when it challenges our own perspective can be hard, but doing so reduces the risk of harm to others. If we truly want to reduce harm to families in pregnancy and birth never should it be about the experience of the caregiver, of their personal beliefs or what it brings to them, but always of that family and what they need to have a positive maternity journey.

This brings me to what I mentioned before the aspect of birth that has been a personal struggle for me. That some have tried to silence me and others concerning our stories suggesting that they bring fear to others and can then cause them to have a negative birth experience. In reality when we listen to women and families often they will voice that they wish there were more honest open conversations about birth and how difficult it can be, also the complexity and impact it can have emotionally. Of course, I'm not saying here that we sit down with every pregnant woman and extoll the intimate details of how birth can be traumatic. We do however owe families the right to have honest open conversations that explore choice, risk, complexity and what matters to them. When we do so we give them the ability to consider what can help them if birth does become a challenging situation. Knowledge is powerful and allows for feeling informed, prepared and able to adapt should this be needed. The truth is that birth is sometimes traumatic and we owe it to families to not hide this but instead be open to hearing why and in turn how we can prevent this for others.

The many faces of birth

So the truth is that birth has many faces and no one situation prevails, it is as individual to each woman, baby and family as a fingerprint. Birth can be very straightforward but it can also be very complicated so providing care and support while respecting individual choice can be challenging.

What are some of the faces of birth? One is the physiological side of birth which we hear so much about. When I trained as a Birth Buddy I learned so much about the human body, its ability to birth and how as women we can help support our bodies, hormones and instincts during the stages of labouring and birth. I truly believe that giving birth can be a wonderful, momentous, truly beautiful event during which a woman can birth her baby safely. In fact, women have been doing exactly that for thousands of years. However, working with women and families who have experienced birth trauma I also see that we must be cautious. Why?

When birth goes well and is the experience a woman hoped for it is amazing. However, we hear women say that when things in birth take a different journey from the one they had envisioned they have struggled and felt like a failure. When her baby comes early, or labour becomes complicated, when coping strategies haven't worked or when a woman hasn't been able to give birth vaginally or has required interventions she may feel her body has failed.

I have personally heard many women voice that they felt let down, that the reality of birth wasn't explained to them and that they felt unprepared and almost lulled into a false sense of security believing that their birth would go to plan if they just believed it and that nature would do the rest. This however isn't always the reality, birth sometimes takes a different turn. Sometimes there are medical complications or emergencies. Sometimes there are other health issues in a woman or her baby meaning that her birth becomes complex.

When a woman doesn't have the birth she wanted then thoughts like 'what's wrong with me' or 'Why did I fail', 'What did I do wrong' or 'I regret my birth' can bring much distress. For some women, it can result in a feeling of despair and sometimes trauma.

So how do we support women but also at the same time not give an unrealistic view of birth? The key here is knowledge that is evidence-based but also realistic and takes into account each woman's wishes and choices as well as her history, previous births, and physical and emotional health. It means honest open conversations about what may happen and how they will or can be supported. It means awareness that the complexity of birth may also limit choices for some and will require more support.

It is also important that we never put one form of birth on a pedestal as the ultimate to be achieved and as a sort of goal or prize to be attained. Why are women that have laboured for hours, attempting to birth vaginally but going on to have interventions feeling like failures? In fact, why does any woman who has birthed a baby feel like a failure? When did it happen that one way of birth equals success and another failure?

A woman I supported a few years ago contacted me for support after going on a Facebook page where women were discussing the length of their labours and competing with each other on how long they laboured before they accepted any pain relief. The woman in question had suffered a very long labour, then an episiotomy, then forceps, then a caesarean because her baby was firmly wedged and in distress. She had reached out to me seeking support because while at first, she had been happy about her birth, she had now begun to feel a failure for having accepted pain relief during her difficult labour, for not having been 'strong enough' to manage without and for then having a caesarean. It was so hard to see her berate herself because of what she felt was a failure on her part to birth her baby the 'right way' based on the opinions of others. Something sadly I hear echoed time and time again.

Women are then often also let down after birth. When birth hasn't gone as planned women are told, 'You have a healthy baby, that's all that matters' but as we have seen this is not true. Birth has a profound effect on a woman and her family and there must be time for reflection after. With so much emphasis on the birth itself, there can be little time given to thinking about after and how this has impacted a woman. Emotionally it can take time to process birth, so time spent with a woman reflecting on her birth can be invaluable, it can lead to conversations that give a safe space to talk through how she feels and anything she may be struggling with. Especially where birth has been traumatic is it important that it is acknowledged and support offered.

Reflecting on difficult and good experiences is important too for healthcare services as it enables learning what helps to make the maternity journey positive and helps improve the care given. It helps to see where improvement is needed and what it is like to be a family using the services provided.

This brings me to another face of birth, the medical side and in particular those who care for women in birth. Maternity staff often come in for a lot of criticism. Sometimes this is justified, but many are trying hard under very difficult circumstances to provide care in birth that is kind, compassionate and patient centred.

I'm not a midwife or an obstetrician but having spent many hours with those that are I know that being responsible for the safe birth of a baby is a heavy responsibility. No one wants anything to go wrong or a woman or her baby to suffer any harm. However birth can be risky and unpredictable and so in the hast to make it as safe as possible it has in many ways become very medicalised.

Rather than risk injury or the death of a woman or her baby, doctors or midwives will edge on the side of caution. Having procedures and policies in place makes staff feel safe and processing medical training they may see things from a very different angle to the family they are caring for. Add into this the risk of litigation when things do go wrong and it can be a mix that doesn't allow for much movement. It can also be hard to support a woman who although making an informed choice may seem to go against the very medical guidelines that have been set in place to keep her safe. As a result, many women voice that the way they wished to birth has been lost in a sea of policies, with choice gone, and a loss of feeling in control. Of course, for some, this has meant the saving of their life or that of their baby, however for others it has meant they haven't had the birth experience they wanted, had medical interventions they didn't want or didn't understand and have felt coerced or traumatised as a result.

As we have said no one wants anything to go wrong. This leads to the question, how far do we feel women should be able to 'choose' how they give birth? What if they wish to birth a certain way but there is no medical need or it may increase risk?

There may be no clear answer to this and this is where the waters become muddy. It is true that a woman has the choice and control over her own body and baby., but also those caring for her have a responsibility to keep her and her baby safe. Informed choice must truly be that, an informed choice. This is where working together with families is vital as equals in their care and planning. Those caring for women need to take the time to discuss any medical interventions and why they are being suggested. Especially should this be true for women and families who may struggle to access information due to social, cultural, language or other difficulties. Genuine communication is the key. Finding out what her choices are, and why she has chosen certain things. Looking at a woman as a whole person with her own thoughts, ideas, needs, wants and desires. There are so many aspects to birth that include culture or beliefs, that can be spiritual, religious, personal and diverse. This is very challenging and may seem impossible to achieve, but only by doing so can correct information and support be given that relates to that woman and her circumstances.

It can be easy to protest that policies don't allow for choice or we don't understand why a woman may take a certain risk or request an intervention we may feel is not needed but it is good to challenge our knowledge and seek to always learn more to improve the care given. Fear of litigation is very real, however, that fear can lead to leaving no room for choice, movement or consideration of individual requests.

Language matters too in how we address families. Families are diverse and unique. Some may have requests about the use of correct pronouns or how they wish to be referred to within the context of their maternity journey. Wherever possible supporting this on the maternity journey and how this relates to a positive experience can help reduce harm and trauma. I have been told things over the years that have been said to women that have caused me to shrink back in horror. From being told 'they are lazy, harming their baby, selfish, a failure' and more, to my own experience of being called 'pathetic and needy'. Language can be powerful, we have all heard the saying 'The tongue is sharper than a two-edged sword'. Language can harm, wound, tear up and discourage or it can build up, heal and bring comfort and encouragement. I have spoken to so many families where the things said to them have caused so much harm, it has rung in their ears for years inflicting pain every time they are recalled. There have been many campaigns to address language used in pregnancy and birth that have resulted in great improvements. Something that can be a continued reflection for us all.

Another important area is consent. No matter what the situation it is very important that a woman gives consent. I've lost count of the number of women who have voiced that they had procedures done to them during birth that they did not consent to or that felt they had no choice but to allow. Communicating why, and making sure that a woman fully understands and consents to anything done to her cannot be overly stated. I have had women voice that it has felt like they were violated and abused in the most intimate ways when consent was ignored, even likening it to rape. We have an obligation to reduce trauma by being respectful of women's bodies and the importance of the need to gain their consent. Trauma-informed care comes from the basis that we do not always know what women have experienced and as such consent is vital in keeping them emotionally safe.

Supportive antenatal education

Antenatal education also plays a vital role in helping reduce trauma and support families in birth. Sadly many families have voiced that they felt their antenatal classes left them feeling unprepared for the reality of birth.

Antenatal education has the potential to allow space for the sharing of information that informs, supports and allows for honest reflection on what birth can mean. It can allow for discussions for options in birth if plans change, or if interventions are needed and how this can be supported. Also the explanation of the roles of the different staff who may care for them and what can be offered to families in practical ways. It can give space to discuss fears or concerns that will not be belittled or downplayed. It can help families to build trust, feel heard and plan their birth in ways that allow for its complexity and doesn't give preference to any one 'truth'.

Antenatal classes should be given in a non-judgemental way, that reflects the complexity of families. It should not be idealist, or unrealistic. Especially should time be given to discussing mental health in pregnancy, birth and after, including what support is available if birth is difficult and how families can access this if needed.

Antenatal care should also be tailored for all, namely it should be available to those who are hopeful of a physiological birth but also those who have a planned caesarean. By openly discussing the complexity of birth we do much to reduce the possibility of birth being traumatic.

Why Kindness and compassion matter.

Kindness as one dictionary defines it is, 'going out of your way to be nice to someone or to show a person you care'. Other definitions say kindness embodies generosity, selflessness and love.

Compassion one dictionary states is, 'caring more about the thoughts and feelings of others than your own', another definition says compassion is, 'a feeling of deep sympathy and sorrow for another who is stricken by misfortune'.

Kindness and compassion are words we hear a lot when discussing care given to families in birth, but are these truly reflected in the care given and the services provided? The truth is kindness and compassion are just as important as the medical care provided, the equipment used, and the policies put in place to protect the safety of mothers and babies.

Poor care that is devoid of kindness and compassion, can leave families feeling vulnerable and even traumatised. The effects can be long-lasting and life-changing. While of course, it matters the medical care given, without it being enveloped in kindness and compassion it can unknowingly cause harm to those being cared for. Simple acts of kindness and showing compassion in dealing with families and also staff with each other can go a long way in making very difficult and sometimes traumatic situations easier to bear.

So how can kindness and compassion be kept at the centre of care? What can individuals and services do to keep kindness and compassion firmly in focus?

Families put their trust in healthcare professionals to help them when they are at their most vulnerable, sometimes even placing their very lives in their hands, this is true in birth. They rely on them not only to give good accurate evidence-based information, and medical care that will keep them and their baby safe, but also that protects them from harm not only physically, but emotionally.

With the pressures of the modern healthcare system, it is easy to lose sight of the simple things, that make a hospital stay easier. Forgotten sometimes are the kind words and the feeling of deep sympathy and sorrow for someone who requires care. Hospital in particular can be a scary place. Away from home, without loved ones around, often in pain or worried about what will happen, women during birth look to those in place to care for them for reassurance and comfort. For many the birth of their baby will be the first time they go into a hospital so feeling safe and cared for with kindness and compassion can go a long way in preventing trauma.

Do families come first?

To reduce birth trauma everyone must work together to build services that have kindness and compassion at its core. It is important that kindness and compassion are the focus of care given in maternity services. This is done in two ways, the culture of maternity units and the personal, inner, values of those that work in maternity services.

It is good for maternity services to reflect on what they are like for both families and the staff that work in them. Does the culture of maternity units allow for kindness and compassion, does it nurture and grow them? Do staff work as a team, all supporting and trusting each other?

Does the culture show that women, babies and families come first? Does the language used reflect that staff care, that they have time for, and want to listen to families and that their thoughts, needs and opinions matter?

Do maternity units allow for families to feedback on their experiences and thoughts, are these valued and appreciated or just token listened to? Is the culture flexible to meet the needs of more complex needs, if a woman or her partner is disabled, or needs help to communicate due to language needs or learning difficulties? Or maybe mental health issues mean a woman needs extra support and understanding.

Is the culture of the maternity unit based on policy, data, paperwork and procedures, is it target driven and what is best for the staff, not women and babies? Does the culture dictate the care given, unyielding to the needs of families, making women feel like they are a burden, bothering staff or too afraid to ask for help?

These can be hard questions to reflect on with so many demands. Combined with a lack of resources, it can feel overwhelming, maybe impossible, to give care that is not only medically good but shows genuine kindness and compassion too. However, it matters because when kindness and compassion are lacking it profoundly affects the experience of birth for the woman and her partner.

To encourage a culture that is focused on kindness and compassion means staff need support. Good communication, praise and feeling valued are vital. Good management is also important. Allowing staff to grow, treating them with respect and making them feel appreciated will help keep the culture in a maternity unit healthy.

It's important too that staff are listened to. I have heard over the years many voice that they have tried to speak up about things that they have felt are wrong or practices that raise concerns, only to be dismissed. Worse than this I have known staff who have been bullied for speaking out, being forced to move roles even hospitals due to how they have been treated. If staff are raising concerns they must be listened to., they are the ones with the families and in the birthing space. Over and over again we hear when investigations are done into poor care in maternity units that staff tried to raise concerns and were ignored. The results are devastating both to staff and families, sometimes the biggest price of all being paid is the loss of a woman or her baby.

Winning the minds and hearts of staff starts with approachable management. Feeling that issues can be raised, ideas can be shared and they have an active role to play in improving services encourages staff and makes hearts swell with pride. Often when managers listen to their staff they will know what the service needs, what families need and how care can be given in a productive but kind and compassionate way. When a culture flourishes, staff will flourish as will the care they give to families.

Personal inner values

The second important part of showing kindness and compassion is an individual's own inner values.

If you care for women during pregnancy and birth ask yourself. Do I see labels or people? Do I take responsibility for my own actions or do I blame the culture? Am I showing kindness to others I work with and the families I care for? Do my actions show that compassion is my focus? How do I view women under my care, are they a privilege or a burden? Does the way I manage or treat work colleagues set an example of kindness? Am I critical and indifferent to the needs of others? What does my language communicate to those I care for and my colleagues? Am I approachable, friendly and adaptable?

These can be hard questions to face. But it is important to look at personal inner values. When everyone maintains their own inner values, if they remember they are accountable for the care they give women. If they keep families at the centre they can make the care given focused on kindness and compassion. If they speak up when they see something is wrong and do all they can to be an example of kindness and compassion then not only do they build a better culture but also safeguard the emotional wellbeing of those they care for. Being aware that while the systems around them may not be doing well in caring for families, they can make a difference on an individual level. Thinking about how they would feel in that person's shoes, about what they would want for their family member needing care, or reflecting again on why they chose to work in maternity services can help to keep inner values on track. Inner values and a healthy culture go hand in hand.

Women over and over again tell us that kindness and compassion matter to them. It may only be small things, saying hello at a reception desk, holding a woman's hand while she undergoes a test, sitting talking with a mother sat by her baby's incubator, fetching a cup of tea for a new father waiting for his loved one to come out of surgery or sometimes just offering a little reassurance and empathy. These small acts can mean so much to a family especially if they are worried, scared and feeling overwhelmed. While we may never know the effect of any kindness shown, that family will remember it for a lifetime.

Especially at difficult times this really does matter. If birth becomes an emergency situation, or a baby is born early or sick. If a family lose their precious baby or a woman is seriously ill then the kindness and compassion shown to them can make the difference at such a difficult time, reducing trauma and helping families to cope.

Thankfully there are many working hard to show real kindness and compassion every day in our maternity units, both in small ways and in making large-scale changes. By working closely with families, listening and sharing ideas we can enable the improvement of services to reflect not only good evidence-based care but kindness and compassion, especially at such a vulnerable time as birth.

Medically the care given to women and babies matters, sometimes it saves lives, however, kindness and compassion matter too. When we listen to women and staff, and show kindness and compassion it improves the culture of our maternity units. It improves care given during pregnancy, birth and after, it helps staff feel appreciated and valued, and women cared for and safe. It means feedback for services that build a good reputation, and give staff praise for all their hard work as well as inner joy for making a difference.

We can prevent birth trauma together.

Birth may indeed have many faces. Teamwork, communication, consent and dignity all play a part.

Women and staff need a good relationship built on trust. This can only happen when there is honesty and when communication is to hear, and not to speak, when consideration is given to each family and their needs. It also means each individual who is surrounding the woman and her family takes personal responsibility for their actions, words and part in the wider system. Improving birth and reducing trauma takes everyone coming together, to hear, to learn, to make a difference. It is a collective approach born out of the desire to keep families safe emotionally as well as medically.

On a personal note, I implore anyone who works with families on the maternity journey to reflect on and hear those who can bear the pain of sharing their stories. It takes a huge amount of sacrifice, courage and the reliving of many painful moments to share experiences that have caused great harm. To those that hear these stories it can be a gift, it can give precious insight, allow space for healing and the potential to improve birth experiences in the future. It allows us to see that if we work together and seek to understand what matters to families we can make birth better for all.

So too failure has no place in birth because no woman fails but only does her best in the circumstances she finds herself in. Birth is not a competition, it isn't the same journey for any two women, in fact for any two babies. Birth is individual, it can be wonderful and breathtaking, and sometimes it can be difficult and heartbreaking but, if women and families are at the centre, are the motive, the reason, the purpose, then everyone will always strive to make every birth the best it can be.

For me so much of my trauma was preventable. It was small things, kindness, compassion, being given a sandwich or the help to visit my baby that would have made a huge difference and could have prevented my journey from being so traumatic. I believe we can prevent so much harm being caused by simply listening to hear, by reflecting on whose experience birth is, by showing kindness and compassion and by letting go of 'our truth' to see the bigger picture, the huge tapestry that is the complexity of birth.

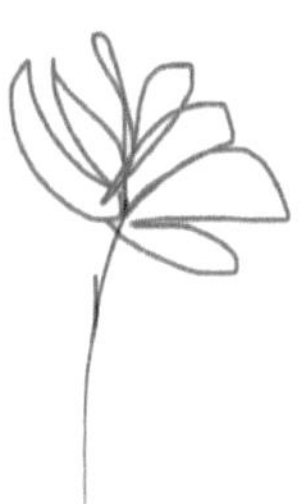

14

AND FINALLY……..

So here you are at the end of the book. I'm not sure where you are on your road to healing. I know however the pain and turmoil that comes with this journey that you did not ask for but was instead forced upon you.

Over the years as I look back there are so many things I wish I could tell the me back when trauma held me so tightly. I see the woman I was before and who I am now. So much has changed both in my life and in me as a person. I wish I could hug the old me who was in pain, who was consumed by guilt and blame. I wish I could whisper to myself that I mattered, that it wasn't my fault, that I was stronger than I believed.

I love looking at photographs. In a world where camera phones and selfies are the thing there's still nothing quite like a real photograph. They say a picture can speak a thousand words, and if you look hard and long enough at those old memories I believe that to be true.

I have a box in my wardrobe containing all my children's memories from locks of hair to tiny baby grows and of course photos. Now and then I open the pretty box and lift out each item so precious and then each album, memories flooding back, some that I had forgotten, others that reminded me of different places and times.

One album is the weeks and months after I had my first daughter. When I look through it's hard to look at the face staring back at me from the pages. My pale face and dark sunken eyes are evidence of the events that had nearly taken both our lives. The photographs clearly show how ill I was physically but they don't tell the whole story, for beneath the pale stricken face lay all the emotional pain of birth trauma. The familiar sting of sadness hits me deep inside because I have so few pictures of my first daughter's early days. Those I do have are a reminder of the events that befell us both and the hurt that followed. It is another loss of birth trauma, one I have grieved many times.

Yet as pick up each album and turn the pages, time passes in months and years and as it does so my heart swells as there is photograph after photograph of my beautiful daughters. My first, tiny and dainty with her big, brown, doe eyes and golden hair. My second, bouncy and happy, with big blue eyes and dark curly hair. As different in looks as they are in personality, and this is true also for the stories of their birth. As I look at all the memories the tears begin to fall and heavy sobs rack my body, because I realise that my babies were happy. Smiles, giggles and laughter light up each page. From feeding the animals at the farm to being pushed on the swings at the park and building sandcastles on the beach.

Those smiles mean so much because I always doubted I was a good mummy. As birth trauma ravaged my mind I believed I was a burden to my family. Some days I even believed my family would be better off without me. Yet as I look at the pictures my heart can see how foolish that was. I was there for my children, doing and giving them everything I could. I loved them with a strong love that nothing could break and it was that love that saved me, that drove me on to get the help I needed no matter what. Despite the pain I felt inside my daughters came first, they were my world and still are. There were days when the impact of trauma was so bad that those simple trips to the park took every bit of energy I had. The smiling faces in those precious photographs remind me how the battle was worth it because to my daughters their mummy was there, holding their hands, cuddling them and loving them completely.

I remember all the days that I worried about how my struggle was affecting them and felt racked with guilt for the things I couldn't do. I was truly seeing things through a trauma lens. Yet the truth was all they needed was my love. My love made sure I was there no matter the battle that raged in my mind. I was there every night to tuck them in bed and there every day at the school gates for them to run into my arms. I was there in the middle of the night when their temperatures raged and there to kiss them better when they scraped their knees. There at every parent's evening and every school assembly. We baked cakes and made dens. I held them in my arms as babies, toddlers and young women, next to my heart, enveloping them in my love.

The photographs showed that my love shone through, through the pain, through the darkness to light up their hearts and give them what they needed which was my love. Then as I have watched them grow into young women they are everything I dreamed they would be. I am proud beyond words to be their mum, such precious gifts that I have been blessed with. This has been my final destination of healing, to love and be loved, to see my children build lives of their own and to now also have the gift of being Nanna! I am so very glad that I fought trauma's grip that tried to take all this from me, that tired to make me believe the lies it told.

Every time I look at those photographs they are hours well spent because they help me remember despite everything I was a good mummy – after all.

So in my final words, one mother's heart to another, don't let birth trauma win. Envelope yourself in the smiles of your children, in the warmth of their embrace. Know that you are the very thing they need, regardless of the struggles you may face. That love indeed can endure all things, that hope is stronger than fear, and that healing is possible for you, as it was for me.

I can't go back and hold the woman with the pale sunken face in those photographs, but I can reach out to you, I can whisper to you the things I wish I had heard. I can tell you that healing from birth trauma is a road you can travel, I'm there, right by your side, along with so many others who also have healed beyond birth trauma. I hope this book has given you even the smallest moment of light to guide you on your way.

All my love
Emma Jane x

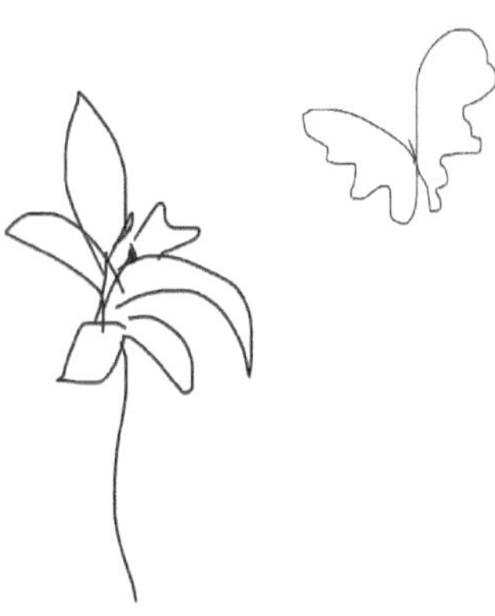

THANK YOU

I would like to thank my husband for putting up with me while I poured my heart out in this book, for helping me with all the tech, and for being my biggest advocate.

My deepest gratitude as always goes to the women who allowed me to use their quotes, and shared with me their pain and hopes on their journey of healing.

To the many many families that I have come to know over the years that have inspired me, trusted me and shared with me their most vulnerable thoughts and moving stories. I never take for granted how hard it is to share your experiences and yet such a privilege to hear them.

To the healthcare professionals who seek to hear our stories, to know that birth trauma matters, that look in themselves to try to bring about change. Who continue to offer friendship and who through their actions and words built trust and belief in me again that prevention of birth trauma is possible.

Thank you x

Don't forget you can find me at Unfoldyourwings.co.uk

NOTES & DOODLES

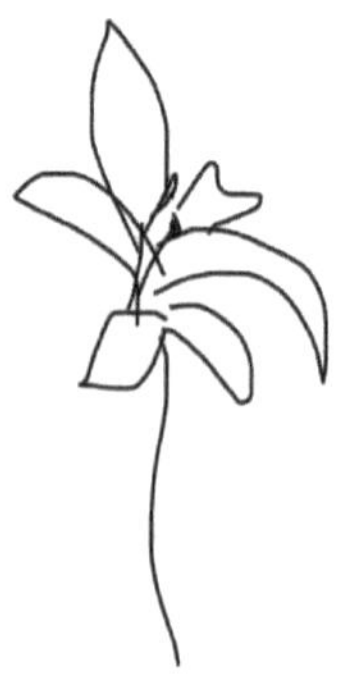

NOTES & DOODLES

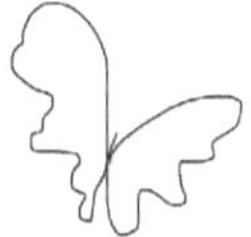

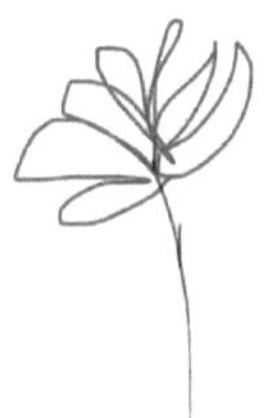